MW01251234

Coping With Fatigue

Coping With Fatigue

By Claude R. Maranda

Four Seasons Publishers
Titusville, FL

Coping With Fatigue

For information contact: Four Seasons Publishers
P.O.Box 51, Titusville, FL 32781

PRINTING HISTORY
First Printing 2001

ISBN 1-891929-52-6

PRINTED IN THE UNITED STATES OF AMERICA
1 2 3 4 5 6 7 8 9 10

TABLE OF CONTENTS

INTRODUCTION

In adult medical practice, fatigue is one of the most common complaints that bedevils the family physician. Sick or healthy, young or old, rich or poor, the average mortal will be victimized by excessive fatigue at some point in his life. Victimized because the average mortal is not just preoccupied with the struggle for survival, he is obsessed with the lure of success, winning at any cost. The performance constraints imposed by a sense of fatigue are a universal encumbrance that frustrate the overachiever, the ambitious, the harried working mother and the stressed-out blue-collar worker who is just trying to make ends meet. Fatigue is endemic, pervasive, and a most serious potential detraction from the pure enjoyment of life. In short, it can drain away the life-blood of simple happiness, not to mention productivity and success.

To realize the significance of a state of fatigue, imagine how your life would be different if the natural limitations imposed by tiredness were eliminated. Boundless energy, the harnessing of "wasted" time (resting and sleeping) and the perpetual feeling of freshness and vitality would revolutionize every aspect of your life. Obviously, this fantasy is impossible; nevertheless, a partial recuperation in this area could be highly profitable.

This book rests its foundation on the following propositions: fatigue is a formidable natural constraint, it can be understood, it can be manipulated, it can be tamed and a thoughtful respect for its biological raison d'etre can be an important determinant of a happy life. Simply accept the possibility and enjoy the journey. We will explore the very nature of the state of fatigue and its physiological mechanisms to devise rewarding strategies to control it.

If you have any skeptical hesitations about the importance of this subject, take a long reflective pause. There is no doubt that the new millennium with its quickening pace of life, its deluge of instantaneous information, its menu of bewildering choices and its deepening complexities at all levels of human endeavour will serve us with a luxuriant lifestyle that will pit the need to overperform against the natural biological restraints of our organism. The risk of rampant chronic fatigue is very high. Fortunately the end-result of this impending maladaptation is entirely preventable. Read on.

For those of you who suffer from disabling fatigue, either because of an illness or an unbalanced lifestyle, a fatigue that is overwhelming and demoralizing, take heart. There are solutions. If you follow the recommendations contained in this book, you will be, at the very least, improved and, in some cases, I daresay, immeasurably better off than you would have been without your current affliction. You are familiar with the oft-repeated saying: "when given a lemon make lemonade." In the case of chronic fatigue it is possible to so effectively manage the problem that the critical adjustments in your life will shower you with benefits much beyond the restrictions that your fatigue ever imposed on you and be a happier more productive human being in the process. The motivational forces unleashed by the problem at hand can magically transform your whole being. Yes, you can regenerate a wonderful life by overcoming a handicap and fine-tuning every aspect of your life.

CHAPTER 1
THE NATURE OF FATIGUE

We are so busy dashing about, so well acquainted with the sensation of fatigue that, like an entrenched habit, we take it for granted and rarely concern ourselves with its deep biological meaning. When was the last time you questioned yourself about the physiological dynamics of fatigue, its role in modulating biological systems and its mission of protecting vital functions of our organism? Have you ever perceived fatigue as anything other than good old-fashioned plain tiredness? What is it? Where is it? What causes it and what mediates it? What changes it? Is it the same for everybody? What is its role, if any, in the proper functioning of my body and mind? Why am I feeling so much of it? These questions could go on and on. The answers are not all obtainable, but there is enough known on which to base a rational approach to its alleviation.

A DEFINITION OF FATIGUE

The common description of fatigue is that of a sense of weariness or tiredness where your will to, or your capacity to, perform work is diminished. You are less inclined to continue whatever led to a state of fatigue, your efforts diminish in frequency, intensity and duration and you feel a powerful urge to rest or sleep with the expectation that a period of rest will restore your full baseline sense of vitality. The actual sensation of weariness is diffuse and ill-defined. It pervades your mind and your body equally, with no clear demarcation between them.

The dictionary defines fatigue as a sense of weariness after exertion or hard work; a condition of cells, tissues or organs which, as a result of excessive activity, temporarily lose their power to respond to further stimulation; a condition of a material such as a metal causing loss of elasticity and tendency to fracture after long or repeated stress, even though the stress may be less than that which would cause failure under static conditions.

The world literature paints a different hue of the state of fatigue that reflects its many variations in real life. Great writers have bequeathed to us innumerable synonyms of the word to enrich its meaning and to expose its multifaceted personality. Table 1.1 lists some of the words commonly used as alternatives to denote slightly divergent meanings.

Dr. Claude R. Maranda

TABLE 1.1
SYNONYMS OF FATIGUE

tiredness	enfeebled
weariness	burned
exhaustion	played out
prostration	knocked flat
lassitude	floored
debility	leveled
enervation	powerless
lethargy	lazy
listlessness	frailty
jaded	lack of energy
fagged	lack of vitality
done	sickliness
done in	impaired
dead beat	devitalized
dog tired	incapacitated
whacked	sluggishness
bushed	inertia
knackered	inactivity
pooped	slowness
dead	sloth
ready to drop	torpor
sapped	lifelessness
languor	languidness
worn	apathy
worn out	passivity
spent	somnolence
taxed	narcosis
washed out	spiritless
weak	unenergetic
collapse	lifeless
faintness	indolent
asthenia	heavy

3

used up
depleted
consumed
dissipation

limp
sleepy
drowsy

Certain themes stand out. The concepts of inadequacy of energy supplies (depletion, drained, sapped, burned out, spent, used up etc), diminished performance (ready to drop, inertia, weak, slow, lethargy, impaired, sluggishness etc), and a state of enfeeblement (limp, heavy, devitalized, debility, asthenia, prostration, powerless etc) stand out as the dominant ones.

These derivations of the meaning of fatigue provide a deeper knowledge (fed by centuries of human experience) of the biological nature of the sense of fatigue. They tell us that fatigue is inherently linked to the energy production facilities of the human body, that fatigue is a product of the natural limits of energy generation and that its presence is a consequence of approaching these limits: diminished performance and a state of enfeeblement. This is not an immaterial observation. It actually reaches down to the most elemental and critical areas of animal biology. Ponder, for a minute, the consequences of a state of diminished performance and weakness in the context of surviving in a treacherous environment. It is quite clear that they would confer a crippling disadvantage in the quest for survival. Fatigue is at the core of human subsistence and is, therefore, a most crucial issue.

To broaden our understanding of fatigue, it is useful to scrutinize how the term has been applied in various fields (physics, biology, psychology) to gain deeper insight into its workings.

METAL FATIGUE

Metal fatigue refers to a **weakened state** in a metal (crystalline solid) resulting from repeated stresses such as cyclical loading, vibrations, mechanical loading (bending back and forth), sheer stress (torsion), thermal stress (contraction and expansion), contact stress (sliding against), corrosive stress and so on. The state of fatigue can lead to a sudden rupture of the metal triggered by a physical stress much less intense than it would have taken at the outset in a perfectly sound unfatigued state. The fatigued solid is thus in an enfeebled state vulnerable to a complete collapse as the result of an ongoing stress.

The mechanism of metal fatigue in its simplest form is that of an initial crack nucleation (a rupture of the crystalline lattice of the solid) which progressively propagates by an enlarging rift. The uncracked portion of the metal adjacent to the propagating crack becomes smaller in cross-section and progressively weaker. Any imperfection in the metal will favor progressive expansion of the fracture. Metal fatigue is therefore a diminishment of its essential function of tensile strength up to its ultimate failure (rupture) if the inciting stress goes unabated.

The prevention of metal fatigue can be enhanced by eliminating defects in the material, avoiding stress concentrations, diversifying stress types, combining metals to improve tensile strength (alloys) and altering the strength of bonding at the atomic level by manipulating the temperatures at which the metals are forged. As will be evident in future chapters, these inorganic strategies are applicable to biological systems.

MUSCULAR FATIGUE

Perhaps the type of fatigue the reader will be most familiar with is muscular fatigue. A muscle cell's essential function is contraction, thus shortening and approximating whatever structures are attached to either end. By rhythmically contracting and relaxing, muscles can effect posturing of the body and carry out locomotion. This capacity of contraction and shortening is brought about by a series of filament lattices that actuate shortening by sliding along one another. The whole apparatus of sliding filaments is controlled by a vast array of regulatory proteins, and a variety of minerals, principally calcium. This intense mechanical

5

work requires fuel (sugars, fats, oxygen), as well as regulatory enzymes (ATPase) and generates metabolic end-products such as lactic acid.

Fatigue results in a failure of the muscle to sustain its contractile force or to regain its maximal power after repeated contractions. In other words, it is diminishment in the ability of the muscle cell to contract at its normal proficiency. This fatigue translates into weakness and diminished capacity to walk, run, leap, lift, or even stand.

Fatigue is generated by many different mechanisms: alterations or vitiations of the neuromuscular junction (pre-synaptic and post-synaptic membrane, acetylcholine), of the electrochemical depolarization of the cell membrane (i.e. cooling), of the excitation-contraction coupling (release of intracellular calcium), of the actin-myosin interaction (sliding filaments), depletion of energy stores (glucose, fat, oxygen), accumulation of metabolic end-products (lactic acid), abnormal mitochondrial metabolism and any number of pathological conditions. The essential feature of weakened muscular contractions (fatigue) can be achieved in many different ways. The potential causes of abnormal muscular fatigue are very numerous.

Common muscular fatigue, the one we all experience with prolonged muscular work or unaccustomed exercise, is largely the result of the accumulation of lactic acid within the muscle cell (metabolic waste product). Because the removal of lactic acid from the muscle is slower than its production, it will accumulate under conditions of intense muscular work, causing intracellular acidosis and, consequently, interfering with p^H-sensitive biochemical reactions within the contractile apparatus. Thus, a degradation of contractile function. Thus, muscle fatigue.

MYOCARDIAL FATIGUE

Heart muscle fatigue can serve as a prototypic example of internal organ fatigue. As you can well assume, the heart muscle contractile function is programmed to work continuously at a pre-scribed pace to sustain the circulation. However, like any other biological system, it is genetically programmed to work within pre-set limits. If the organ is forced to work beyond its natural limits, fatigue will set in.

A good example of the consequences of energetic over-reaching is the circumstance where the heart is forced to work intensely, continuously, either by rapid pacing or by working against a resistance load (valvular stenosis). Slowly but surely, contractile function will deteriorate, weaken and will result in an inadequate forward cardiac output. This triggers a set of hemodynamic adjustments resulting in cardiac dilatation and congestive heart failure. Myocardial fatigue will set in motion compensatory mechanisms such as hypertrophy but ongoing overwork will soon overwhelm these compensatory mechanisms and lead to cell death.

The biochemical mechanism of myocardial fatigue is not known but several factors play a role: triggering of apoptosis (programmed cell death), insufficient oxygen supply to meet the enhanced demand, energy production insufficient to meet energy utilization, abnormal intracellular calcium transport (the link between the electrical activity of the cell and its contractile function), diminished depolarization of the cell membrane, ion channel dysfunction and a vicious circle initiated by compensatory adrenergic drive (exacerbates the energy supply/demand imbalance). Regardless of the actual mechanism, myocardial fatigue is a state of diminished work capacity as a result of overwork. Heart failure is the result.

METABOLIC FATIGUE

Metabolic functions, activated by billions of biochemical reactions, are not unlimitedly capacitated given enough fuel or substrate. Quite the contrary. Metabolic pathways operate at finite rates, limited proficiency and do develop fatigue-like features.

An example is diabetes mellitus (sugar diabetes). Individuals who develop insulin-resistance for any reason must produce greater amounts of insulin than normal to maintain sugar levels and sugar metabolism. This incessant, large demand on the insulin-producing cells of the islets of Langherhans (cells in the pancreas that produce insulin) will eventually lead to exhaustion of the machinery that manufactures insulin and ultimately a collapse in production. Compensatory mechanisms (hypertrophy) can sustain the cells temporarily but, unfortunately, it (hypertrophy) carries the seeds of its own demise and the cells nevertheless fail under the unacceptable stress of overwork.

Anorexia nervosa, a psychiatric condition where literal starving deprives metabolic systems of their essential nutrients, will eventually result in a state of fatigue and metabolic failure. Tissues atrophy, malfunction and, if the insult is unremitting, die.

Physiologic maladjustments also lead to fatigue. The best known example is circadian rhythm stress, also known as synchronization stress and jet-lag. In this example, diurnal cycles (24 hours) which are based on cycles of darkness and light are thrown out of kilter by rapid time zone changes and lead to mismatches between "daytime" mental and physical functions and metabolic (hormonal) levels of activity. These mismatches render the traveling person very vulnerable to low-threshold fatigue.

PSYCHOLOGICAL FATIGUE

Psychological fatigue is not an unambiguous entity.. The initial presumption would be to perceive psychological fatigue as a waning of emotional fires and a blunting of their physiological effects. Partly. Psychological fatigue is also a weakening of control, a decline in tolerance to stress and a hypersensitivity to emotional stimuli. Loss of control of the fine equilibrium between stress and stress-reactivity is the key point. Several examples will illustrate this.

Combat fatigue or battle fatigue is a state of emotional dysfunction brought about by excessive stress encountered on the battlefield. Exposure to physical hardship, prolonged exertion and intense conflicting emotions can lead to: (1) hypersensitivity to stimuli such as noises, movements and light accompanied by overactive responses that include involuntary defensive jumping or posturing (startle reactions); (2) hair-trigger irritability progressing even to acts of violence; and (3) sleep disturbances including battle dreams, nightmares and insomnia. Fatigue in this setting is manifested as a decrease in the ability of the afflicted individual to control his emotions.

Addiction battle-fatigue, with its cycles of submissions and capitulations, is another example of psychological fatigue. The addicted casualty can demonstrate signs of fatigue as constant craving gradually grates at his will to resist: as fatigue sets in, control systems weaken and can fail abruptly.

Professional burnout is another familiar example of a form of psychological fatigue. Your obsessive-compulsive Type A personality cultivates a lifestyle of workaholism, denies himself a balance between work and leisure, always pushing for more responsibilities, more successes, shouldering his and everybody else's problems, impelled to walk, talk and eat rapidly, in short, your average burnout candidate jumps on the treadmill first thing in the morning and reluctantly gets off for bedtime. Result: depletion of psychological resources allied to a progressive diminishment in the ability to resist stress. The victim will slip into a state of weariness, indecisiveness, depression, irritability, declining productivity, unreliability, negativity and proneness to substance abuse. As fatigue sets in, compensatory mechanisms kick in only to exacerbate the downward spiral.

GENERAL FATIGUE

General fatigue is an inner sense of an ill-defined sluggishness coupled with a decreased will and/or capacity to continue productive work. This state can be reached by any number of different paths but primarily by muscular exertion, prolonged cerebration or by emotional taxing. All three, individually or in any combination, can lead to a state of fatigue. Psychological factors play an important modulating role because perception can significantly change the threshold at which motivation and volition deteriorate. The consequences of general fatigue include a composite of an objective and subjective inadequacy and a free-floating aversion to continuing the tasks at hand.

A SYNTHESIS: THE NATURE OF FATIGUE

From the overview of different forms of fatigue, one can cull certain key elements characteristic of fatigue. Table 1.2 schematizes its skeletal elements.

As is evident from the schema, fatigue is a progressive weakening and diminishment of performance when work rate extends beyond the working entity's natural capacity. This imbalance between supply and demand can be tolerated if temporary and redressed by adequate amounts of rest. Furthermore, this temporary imbalance can be extended by tapping into compensatory mechanisms that can sustain the working machinery for exceptional demands. Presumably the ability to draw on biological support mechanisms for extraordinary circumstances (i.e. running away from a predator, ability to travel long distances to find food) would have provided a survival advantage to the animal and consequently favored by evolution. These back-up compensatory mechanisms unfortunately are doubled-edged. Abuse them and they will lead to energy depletion and biochemical dysfunction that will ultimately threaten the very survival of the cell or organ. There are innumerable examples in the realm of biology or medicine where sustained overwork with overriding of the natural fatigue restraint and the persistent utilization of compensatory mechanisms will lead to cellular disintegration and death.

- Depression: While fatigue is a very frequent accompaniment of depression (in fact it might well be the most common cause of unnatural fatigue) they are not synonymous. What is characteristic of depression is psychomotor retardation (a feeling that every motion and every thought is "weighed down with lead").

- Drowsiness is similar to sleepiness but that soporific feeling may also be the result of metabolic disturbances (high blood sugar, low sodium), drug side-effects, poisonings such as carbon monoxide inhalation, low oxygen levels in blood, severe anemia and an inadequate cerebral circulation. Drowsiness is not always fatigue.

- Laziness is often an outcome of excessive fatigue but generally is more of a "won't do" rather than "can't do." Shortness of breath, a feeling of labored breathing is some-

- times confused with fatigue. Many patients report feeling exhausted by ordinary walking when, in fact, they are short of breath. The diagnostic implications are quite different.

GRADING OF FATIGUE

How fatigued are you? The answer is problematic. Being a poorly-defined inner sensation devoid of easily-measured objective signs, one is left with all the pitfalls of attempting to quantify a subjective matter. Grading is not totally academic. It does help a physician's decision-making based on the "seriousness" of the condition. Throw into the broth neurosis, depression, hypochondriasis and whining and you can understand how complicated it is for a physician to sort out a complaint of general fatigue. There are two traps for the beleaguered doctor: one is to ignore the complaints out of sheer frustration and the other is to over-investigate every mundane grumblings of "being tired." The latter approach is a recipe for bankruptcy (of the system) and all the problems of laboratory false-positives. These falsely abnormal lab results lead to still further expensive and unnecessary demands on the laboratory. It takes patience, experience and wisdom to find the middle road.

Fatigue severity can be graded into four classes:

Class I: normal fatigue
Class II: mild fatigue
Class III: moderate fatigue
Class IV: severe fatigue

Class I fatigue is determined by averages. It is the frequency and intensity of tiredness that is experienced by 95% of the normal population for any given age group. An estimate of this quantity can only be made through experience.

Class II: mild fatigue is an amount of tiredness which is slightly more than the average of a normal population for activities that are clearly out of the ordinary. For example, walking for hours at a time, playing singles tennis for more than an hour, shopping all day, partying till the wee hours of the morning, moving, travelling, working overtime, frenzied work to meet a deadline, writing an exam and giving a speech. The fatigue is excessive relative to an average, but it is not disabling and the individual is fully recuperated with a good night's sleep.

Class III: moderate fatigue is when ordinary activities are associated with weariness. The lassitude is pervasive, is not resolved by a good night's sleep and is incapacitating. The individual afflicted with low-threshold fatigue cannot cope with a normal, average lifestyle. He may not be able to hold a full-time job, sports are out of the question, and social activities are severely curtailed.

Class IV: This most serious degree of fatigue is at a level of total exhaustion where even inactivity and constant rest will not resolve it. Exhaustion without doing anything describes it best. This severity of fatigue is most often associated with brutally debilitating diseases and the end-stage of any organ failure, i.e. congestive heart failure.

A semi-quantitative grading of fatigue facilitates the long-term monitoring of the quality of life of the fatigue-sufferer and helps in judging when it makes sense to initiate expensive investigations.

CHAPTER 2
A PHYSIOLOGICAL MODEL OF FATIGUE: THE REGULATOR OF HUMAN WORK OUTPUT

Man and beast do not roam the earth with an electrical plug on their backside to provide motive power. A biological unit must be self-sufficient and generate its own energy. The human body does that with an elaborate biochemical furnace. This furnace can convert primary foodstuffs in energy-rich chemicals that the organism uses to fuel the working machinery. Every cell in the body has its own furnace.

HOW THE BODY GENERATES ENERGY

The simplest way to gain an understanding of the process of energy generation and consumption is to fancifully hop onto your favorite dessert (let's make it a sinful cheesecake!) and follow it through its many meanderings and transformations as it becomes converted into a unit of energy.

As the cheesecake is lustfully ingested, it enters the upper gastro-

16

intestinal tract where it is bathed in a rich broth of digestive enzymes which immediately execute their mission of breaking it down to simpler food units, small enough to be absorbed by the mucosal lining of the gut. What is indigestible (e.g. fibers) is transported along to its final destination of bodily excretion via the colon. The cheesecake, which has been dismantled into its basic constituents of carbohydrates, proteins, fat molecules, vitamins and minerals is now flowing to the liver via the portal veins that drain the gastro-intestinal tract. The liver filters, moulds, stores and repackages the various nutrients to make them suitable for delivery to every corner of the body. It acts like a post office where, from a central hub, the packages of nutrients are redirected to their final destination, the cell.

The cell is designed to recognize its nutrients. With specific receptors on its cell membrane, it is capable of latching onto the foodstuffs in the perfusing blood. When a nutrient is seized by the receptor, it is transported into the cell for distribution along the many way-stations of energy production. These include the protoplasm (the cellular gel that contains enzymes and complex biochemical structures), mitochondria (small bodies that are factories for the production of high-energy ATP), vesicles that are responsible for a variety of metabolic processes and the endoplasmic reticulum (a network of interconnected, closed membrane vesicles) whose most important function is the synthesis of membrane lipids and proteins.

Energy production is highly complex. It is primarily generated by rupturing the electrical bond between atoms. Atoms such as carbon, oxygen, hydrogen, sulfate, phosphate have variable electronic bonds which release their potential energy where disengaged. Glucose and fatty acids, the main molecules that were derived from our initial cheesecake are now within the cell to supply energy. Each molecule is degraded. Through a series of biochemical transformations of the glucose and fatty acids, energy is continually released and harnessed. Harnessing the released energy (potential energy) comes from the formation of ATP (adenosine triphosphate). This product can be considered the universal currency of cellular energy transactions. It is so, because whenever energy is required, ATP is hydrolyzed or "broken up" to release one of its three phosphate atoms. Thus ATP becomes ADP (adenosine diphosphate) + P. This electronic rupture generates enormous amounts of energy that will power essential cellular functions. Some of these include the energy to establish and maintain concentration gradients of various molecules across cell membranes, creating and sustaining electrochemical gradients across these same membranes (exemplified by $Na+$ and $K+$ gradients which are fundamental to neural and muscular conductance), the beating of cilia, the contraction of muscles and in a multitude of biochemical pathways including the synthesis of nucleic acids (DNA) and proteins from amino acids and nucleotides.

ATP needs to be regularly regenerated through the chemical breakdown of foodstuffs with the concert of oxygen and in this fashion, keep the whole metabolic machinery humming.

As is evident from the aforegoing discussion, energy production is an extremely complex and long-winded process. These features make it vulnerable to breakdown; any dysfunction, at any stage of this prolonged process, can lead to diminished performance, which is the essence of fatigue. If we return to the cheesecake for a minute and follow its intricate route, we can plot out all the points of possible dysfunction and thus recognize the potential causes of fatigue. For example, a state of fatigue could result from:

♦ inability to swallow the cheesecake as a result of a stroke
♦ absent or insufficient digestive enzymes as in pancreatic insufficiency
♦ ineffective absorption from the gastro-intestinal mucosa (lining) as in a mal-absorption syndrome
♦ hepatic (liver) insufficiency as in alcoholic cirrhosis of the liver
♦ circulatory deficiency with an insufficient delivery of food stuffs
♦ cellular receptor malfunction making it unable to latch onto nutrients

- enzyme deficiencies, usually genetically-transmitted (here there are literally thousands of syndromes)
- mitochondrial dysfunction, either due to intoxication or a genetically-transmitted abnormality, such as in some muscle diseases
- abnormalities in the programming of amino acid sequencing of various proteins
- deficiencies of vitamins and minerals for any reason
- insufficiency of oxygen for any reason
- malfunction of regulatory proteins for any reason (could be genetic or acquired through disease processes)
- insufficient ATP generation for any reason

The point to be emphasized is that fatigue is an end-product of a myriad of possible malfunctions of the energy production apparatus.

Another important concept in the physiology of fatigue is the proposition that fatigue is a natural consequence of cellular metabolic overreaching. In other words, it is a consequence of too much demand for the available supply. The biochemical furnace that animates every cell of the body has finite limits. It is genetically programmed to work within certain boundaries. This is why a muscle can only do so much contracting, a gland produces only so many hormones and a renal tubular cell only pumps so many electrolytes. There are clear biological limits to all cellular work and fatigue is the sign post. It yells loud and clear: slow down or stop because you are going beyond the natural limits of that particular function.

THE PHYSIOLOGY OF ORGAN FATIGUE

The exact mechanism of most forms of fatigue is not understood. Its consequences, however, are readily observable. A muscle can be shown to decay in contractile performance with repeated stimulation. It is clear that this diminished performance can be caused by many different mechanisms. Almost any malfunction of any portion of the working apparatus or an excess of work can lead to decay in function or fatigue. For example, in working muscles, one can observe fatigue when:

◆ fuels are insufficient (sugars, fat, oxygen, creatine phosphate, ATP)
◆ essential biochemical constituents are deficient (calcium, enzymes, regulatory proteins, phosphates)
◆ accumulation of metabolic end-products (lactic acid)
◆ diminished neurotransmission (depletion of acetylcholine at the neuromuscular plate or receptor malfunction)
◆ diminished membrane electrical activity
◆ mitochondrial abnormalities

It does seem reasonable to conclude that fatigue is not physiologically unique but is a consequence of many types of homeostatic breaches.

How is the information (the presence of fatigue in a tissue or an organ) relayed to the brain for integration with data received from other areas of the body, i.e. other fatigued organs, emotional centers, cognitive centers, consciousness)? Primarily via the peripheral nervous system (sensory nerves, i.e. pain) or the autonomic nervous system (sympathetic, parasympathetic) and, to a much lesser extent, hormonal (either systemic or local). These conduits of information channel a continuous stream of "intelligence" to the brain for integration. The central nervous system (the brain) is then the master receiver of all relevant information and the data "cruncher" to eventually activate the neural regulatory structures to restore homeostasis.

While fatigue signals either distress in a tissue or an imbalance between energy demand and supply, it does not lead to a necessary loss of activity. A cell, an organ, or the whole body, can persevere with a state of fatigue when it has to. This capacity is essential for survival. It is doubtful that any life form could have endured evolution without this ability to continue working in spite of fatigue. This perseverance comes about by the activation of compensatory mechanisms. Compensatory mechanisms that help sustain the work output of an organ for exceptional demands are as

varied as the actual physiological mechanisms of fatigue:
- increased supply of fuel
- hypertrophy (increased mass)
- enhanced circulation and delivery of oxygen, shift in the oxygen-dissociation curve making more oxygen available
- increased rate of waste disposal
- alterations in enzyme levels
- switching of types of fuel for greater efficiency
- hormonal stimulation to enhance energy supplies or accelerate biochemical reactions
- recruitment of working units
- alterations in local hormonal concentrations (kinins, prostaglandins, tissue factors etc)
- inflammation
- neuropeptides
- organ-specific or tissue-specific systems
- slower operating rate

These support mechanisms are generally harmful when overused and therefore of only practical value to meet short-term exceptional needs.

The toxic effects of sustained compensatory mechanisms are well documented but poorly understood. Conceptually, they can be interpreted as leading to a state of profound energy depletion, leaving inadequate supplies to maintain the structural integrity or the biochemical stability of the tissue. This profound energy depletion will lead to cellular disintegration and, ultimately, death. In some tissues (myocardium) apoptosis (programmed cell death) is thought to be a mediator of cell demise under the conditions of inadequate energy supplies to maintain the resting homeostasis of cellular structure. The fundamental biological message is that the operative specifications of an organ are set by nature via genetic programming and must be respected. This natural law applies across the board. Fatigue is a marker of the encroachment on these natural limits.

THE PHYSIOLOGY OF GLOBAL FATIGUE

In this area of human or animal physiology there is a serious deficiency of information. In fact, the word "fatigue" is hardly indexed in any textbook of medicine, biology, physiology, psychology and other less directly-related sciences. The absence of solid scientific data forces us to speculate and construct models with the best available information.

Several logical extrapolations flow from available knowledge of neurobiology. Firstly, only the central nervous system is equipped for the perception of general fatigue. Secondly, as all neurobiological functions are cell-based, one can confidently conclude that a center for fatigue processing must exist either as a cluster of nerve cells (nucleus) or a network of interconnecting neurons. Thirdly, this fatigue center or nucleus, as a result of its varied sources of information and its influence on so many other functions of the central nervous system, must be fully connected, both afferently (into) and efferently (outgoing) to almost every other important area of the central and peripheral nervous system, the autonomic nervous system, neuro-endocrine system (pituitary gland) and probably every organ of the body.

Table 2.1 schematizes the functional anatomy of a neural center for fatigue.

The precise location of a fatigue nucleus or neural network is unknown. The nature of its interaction with other neural centers is also unknown but one could speculate that it is primarily comprised of inhibitory neurons. This is based on the observation that most consequences of fatigue are a diminishment of volitional and vegetative functions of the central nervous system: a diminishment of consciousness, will, motivation, happiness, respiration, circulation (blood pressure) etc.

If we follow the same logical track, one could hypothesize that if nature "installed" such an inhibitory center, there had to be important survival advantages for its "acceptance" as an evolutionary acquisition. Why? The best explanation is the proposition that this inhibitory function evolved to protect the organism against overwork and developing severe energy imbalances that could threaten the integrity of the organism. It is highly probable, therefore, that fatigue plays a vital protective function whose mission is to regulate the equilibrium between energy supply and energy consumption.

TABLE 2.1
FUNCTIONAL ANATOMY OF GENERAL FATIGUE

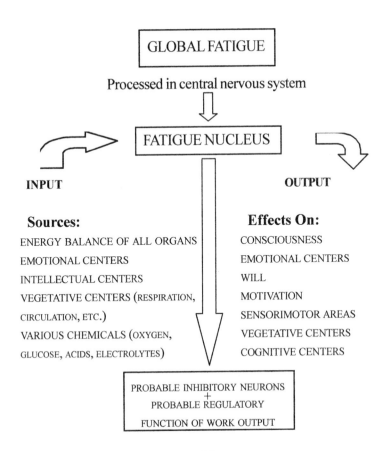

GLOBAL FATIGUE

Processed in central nervous system

FATIGUE NUCLEUS

INPUT

OUTPUT

Sources:

ENERGY BALANCE OF ALL ORGANS

EMOTIONAL CENTERS

INTELLECTUAL CENTERS

VEGETATIVE CENTERS (RESPIRATION, CIRCULATION, ETC.)

VARIOUS CHEMICALS (OXYGEN, GLUCOSE, ACIDS, ELECTROLYTES)

Effects On:

CONSCIOUSNESS

EMOTIONAL CENTERS

WILL

MOTIVATION

SENSORIMOTOR AREAS

VEGETATIVE CENTERS

COGNITIVE CENTERS

PROBABLE INHIBITORY NEURONS
+
PROBABLE REGULATORY
FUNCTION OF WORK OUTPUT

One final assumption. Since fatigue is neurally-based, its cellular physiology is almost certainly identical to all other neurons of the central nervous system: electrochemical membrane conductance by cyclically polarizing and depolarizing and cell-to-cell communication either via electrical synapses (cell-to-cell connection) or via neurochemical transmission in chemical synapses. These neurons would thus obey all the biological laws of neural function, a summary of which is beyond the scope of this book.

CHAPTER 3
THE BIOLOGICAL ROLE OF FATIGUE
AND ITS CONSEQUENCES

As is becoming clearer, fatigue is not simply the passive consequence of an inadequate physiology erecting meaningless barriers
to organ performance. It is clearly a wondrously well-orchestrated
regulatory mechanism that fosters a proper equilibrium between
the everyday needs for survival and the natural specifications of
the biological unit. Its primary tool is inhibition of critical areas of
the brain to slow or halt energy consumption. Failure to respect
the imperatives signalled by fatigue leads to cellular disintegration.

Table 3.1 sketches an overview of the fatigue model.

The fundamental thrust of the model is that there is a central
nervous system monitoring device (fatigue nucleus) that processes
incoming data from every nook and cranny of the body and judges
the biological appropriateness of total energy balance. The incoming data from viscera, cognitive centers and psychological
areas are inseparable. "Hard" or "soft" information are given the

same biological respect.

If the organism encroaches on or exceeds its natural energy limits, the fatigue nucleus will trigger inhibitory impulses to the main neurological engines of action. Alertness is dimmed, will is weakened, aversion is recruited and a demotivating depression sets in. For good reason! To restore a healthy homeostatic balance of total body energy consumption.

The model reveals the basic elements of a highly integrated biological restraint system. It lays bare, in all its natural wisdom, how fatigue is not a nuisance or a disadvantage but, actually, an essential breaking system to safeguard the interests of the human body.

CONSEQUENCES OF FATIGUE

Natural fatigue triggers a compulsion to rest after which the body recuperates and returns to a baseline functional status. What if fatigue is unheeded? Generally no problem. Nature has incorporated ample cushioning in its physiological systems to permit temporary over-reaching without damaging the hardware. However, sustained overwork is toxic and will lead to degeneration and disintegration. The adverse consequences of sustained overwork are extremely varied but can be conveniently classified into three main categories:
- pathological effects on organs
- systemic (general, non-specific)
- psychological dysfunction

Dr. Claude R. Maranda

TABLE 3.1
FATIGUE MODEL

INPUTS INTERACTIONS

INTERNAL:
peripheral energy balance
emotional equilibrium
motivational factors
cognitive centers
recuperation factors
vegetative centers

consciousness
will
alertness
sleep
intellectual centers
Sensorimotor areas
brain stem
neuro-endocrine areas
limbic areas (emotions)

External:
nutrients
toxins
radiation
climactic factors
drugs
chemicals

**Global
Fatigue
Nucleus**

OUTPUT

INHIBITORY EFFECTS

will
consciousness
alertness
motivational factors
stimulatory neurons
happiness center

— **INTEGRATED
BIOLOGICAL
RESTRAINT
SYSTEM**

27

EFFECTS OF CHRONIC OVERWORK ON SPECIFIC ORGANS

Cognitive centers (brain):
diminished intellectual performance, concentration, memory and computational power and an increased incidence of mental errors
Emotional centers:
irritability, loss of control of emotions, increased stress-reactivity, more intense negative emotions, lesser positive emotions, depression, professional burnout.
Vegetative centers (autonomic nervous system):
increased heart rate and blood pressure, accelerated respiration, chronic neurasthenic state, vulnerability to vasodepressive syncope (fainting spells)
Bones:
stress fractures, vertebral collapse, osteosclerosis, spurs
Joints:
supporting structures degeneration (ligaments, cartilage, tendons, bursae), degenerative joint disease (osteoarthritis), osteomalacia.

Muscles:
tears, cramps, cell disintegration (myositis, myoglobinuria), myopathy (dysfunction), weakness, hypertrophy (bulking, diminished flexibility, stiffness)
Heart muscle:
diminished exercise performance, congestive heart failure, arrhythmias
Lungs:
respiratory muscle fatigue, respiratory failure, pneumothorax (rupture due to parenchymal fatigue), emphysema
Liver:
fatty liver, cirrhosis
Gall bladder:
hypertrophy, functional ("lazy" gall bladder)
Pancreas:

maldigestion, diabetes mellitus (certain form)

Gastro-intestinal tract:
dyspepsia (indigestion), gaseous distension, constipation, diarrhea, irritable bowel syndrome.

Renal:
dehydration, electrolyte imbalance, renal failure

Urinary tract:
incontinence, retention

Vascular:
aneurysm, dissection, rupture

Metabolism:
metabolic rate decreases

Glandular:
hormonal deficiency

Sexual organs:
impotence, inability to achieve orgasm, infertility

Immunological:
risk of cancer, infections, auto-immune disorders

PSYCHOLOGICAL CONSEQUENCES OF INTRACTABLE FATIGUE

- motivation weakens
- optimism vanishes
- "joie de vivre" (enjoyment of life) dissolves
- happiness dissipates, depression sets in
- control of emotions loosens
- stress-reactivity increases
- patience diminishes
- introversion substitutes for extroversion
- ability to love wanes
- burnout emerges
- passivity seeps in
- appetites dwindle

♦ risk of aberrant behavior (to compensate) increases

SYSTEMIC CONSEQUENCES OF CHRONIC GLOBAL FATIGUE

♦ judgment errors multiply
♦ accidents crop up
♦ general activity, exercise languish
♦ productivity withers
♦ success in life, wealth creation become unachievable
♦ initiative, imagination, creativity wilt
♦ generosity and altruism are abandoned
♦ risk of illness increases, immunity weakens
♦ human relationships suffer
♦ social withdrawal supervenes
♦ marital failure rises
♦ poor weight control occurs
♦ physical beauty (attractiveness) deteriorates
♦ emotional intelligence (overall management skills of life) declines

The adverse effects of ignoring the physiological "pleadings" of fatigue are nothing short of disastrous. Fatigue is not the cause of biological spoilage but a warning signal that is primordial and deadly serious. I do not believe that it is possible to run a successful and happy life without a conscious, protracted effort to manage the unyielding limits of the human body's operative specifications. The intelligence of fatigue management is an essential component of a fruitful journey on earth.

The realization of this simple proposition is straightforward. Look back at your own personal experiences and contrast the quality of life of a typical day or week of suffocating fatigue to one of bouncy, vigorous elan and draw your own conclusions. No contest. There is no substitute for a well-rested, healthy and invigorated lifestyle for the promotion of genuine happiness.

CHAPTER 4
CAUSES OF FATIGUE

The sensation of fatigue is a universal experience. It is inherent in the animal kingdom; in fact, inherent in the whole biological world. There is therefore a natural fatigue that we readily recognize. We instinctively know how it feels and we intuitively know what causes it. We also learn, somewhat spontaneously, how to deal with it: rest and adjust our daily activities to match our natural limits. Problems arise when natural fatigue is neglected or when unnatural fatigue sets in.

Unnatural fatigue bears no direct relationship to any measure of work output and is not mitigated by adequate rest. When dealing with the issue of problematic fatigue, the first step is to differentiate normal from abnormal or natural from unnatural fatigue. The former and the latter require completely different approaches.

Table 4.1 summarizes the differentiating characteristics of both types of fatigue.

31

TABLE 4.1
NATURAL VERSUS UNNATURAL FATIGUE

NATURAL FATIGUE	UNNATURAL FATIGUE
mild	severe
proportionate to energy expenditure	disproportionate to energy expenditure
within range of past experiences	different from past experiences
short-lived (days)	protracted (weeks)
resolved by simple rest	refractory to "sufficient" rest
explicable by natural physiological processes	not explicable by natural processes
present a small fraction of of everyday living	pervasive
generally at end of a normal day	pancyclic (all day)
unobtrusive and easily tolerable	disturbing
increases with age	age-independent
easily overridden	incapacitating
does not affect motivated performance	diminished performance
not very unpleasant	physically painful

CAUSES OF NORMAL FATIGUE

To clearly visualize the causes of natural and unnatural fatigue, it is very useful to conceptualize a working model of any given biological unit or the body as a whole. Table 4.2 illustrates a simple model that can serve as an anchor for the differential diagnosis of all forms of fatigue.

Natural fatigue occurs when work demand is greater than work output capacity. With a perfectly healthy biological engine, fatigue can occur quite normally. Rest restores working capacity and the system can go on perpetually, given the proper balance between work and rest. Evolutionary forces have favored well-equilibrated biological units so that our mere survival to this day is a testimony of the success of the biological machinery as it exists. The body, however, must be capable of responding to natural challenges explaining its broad operating latitude.

Natural fatigue can be exacerbated by a variety of external conditions. The working model in Table 4.2 lists some of the variables that affect the engine or the adequacy of work output. To illustrate how these variables impact on the production of fatigue, we will analyze scenarios that highlight the relationship between natural impediments and the production of fatigue.

Let us imagine a person who has to survive in the wilderenss with a bare minimum of tools and must build a log cabin for shelter. From day to day, that healthy person would go about cutting trees down, paring them, transporting them, shaping them, and building a house step-by-step. This person would eventually settle on a pace of work compatible with his working capacity and respectful of the equilibrium between total energy expenditure and its full restoration by rest. In this way, a sustainable cycle of appropriate pace of work, fatigue and rest would become established.

TABLE 4.2
MODEL OF FATIGUE
FOR THE DIFFERENTIAL DIAGNOSIS

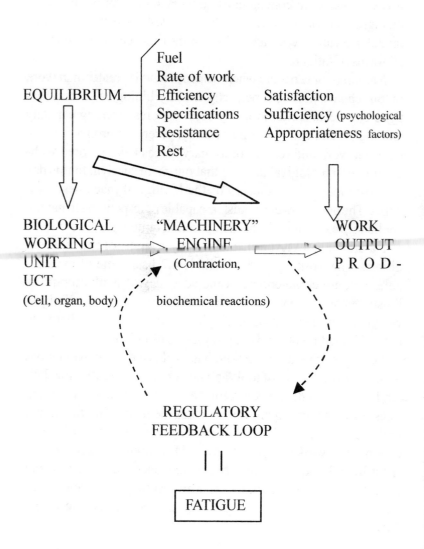

EQUILIBRIUM

Fuel
Rate of work
Efficiency
Specifications
Resistance
Rest

Satisfaction
Sufficiency (psychological
Appropriateness factors)

BIOLOGICAL
WORKING
UNIT
UCT
(Cell, organ, body)

"MACHINERY"
ENGINE
(Contraction,
biochemical reactions)

WORK
OUTPUT
P R O D -

REGULATORY
FEEDBACK LOOP

| |

FATIGUE

An exacerbation of normal fatigue could be induced by a change in any of the modulators of the performance of the engine: availability of fuel, rate of work, rest, resistance to work, specifications of energy expenditure, efficiency of work.

If we would transplant this same person in a high altitude environment, let us say in the Andes at 8,000-10,000 feet, and expected the same work output, severe fatigue would ensue. The decrease in ambient oxygen concentration would diminish the oxygen available to the metabolic machinery and cause a deficiency of energy generation. In this instance, an insufficiency of fuel would aggravate or accelerate the state of fatigue.

Let us now retransplant this same person in a cold, snowy and windy environment and clothe him in the necessary heavy coat and boots. You can imagine how having to carry the heavy clothing and having to slog through snow against a brisk wind would rapidly exhaust our overburdened constructor. The added elements in this scenario represent a form of increased resistance to the work performed and will intensify fatigue.

Still with our same person having to build a log cabin from scratch in different environments, let us now examine how efficiency could change the fatigue equation. Compare one scenario where this individual would have to drag heavy logs from afar on an undulating terrain full of rocks and obstacles with bare hands and the scenario where he would carry the same logs by an alternate route, flat and without obstacles, with the aid of a large well-oiled four-wheeled cart. The latter method is infinitely more efficient and less fatiguing.

The other modulators, rate of work, amount of rest and operating specifications would similarly have a large impact on the production of fatigue. An increased rate of work would disproportionately increase energy expenditure (time premium) and inadequate rest would lead to a cumulative fatigue overhang and exhaust the worker.

Specifications require a more detailed explanation. Every tissue or organ in the animal body is genetically programmed down

to its most intimate details. Every aspect of its structure and its function is as regulated and prescribed as the height, color and shape of
the whole body. The genetic code (endless sequences of nucleic acids
that code for every protein in the body and stored in the nucleus of
every cell of the body) leaves very little room for the environment or
serendipity to weigh in. The upshot of this stark reality is that the
operating capacity of an organ is prescribed by nature, relatively fixed,
and can only vary according to still pre-programmed limits. The biological specifications of any working system are therefore parameters
that must be respected. As already discussed in previous chapters,
the transgression of these natural laws leads to fatigue and, if protracted, to cell death. In this context, one can easily understand how
one person may have a different threshold for fatigue depending on
their genetic make-up. Some fortunate souls are blessed with high
operating capacity (high energy and rarely get tired) and others are
afflicted with low operating capacity (low energy, easy fatigue). Both
are normal but just built differently with divergent specifications.

Natural fatigue is highly influenced by psychological factors. We all
have experienced circumstances where work that we hate leads to
rapid fatigue and work that we love seems to be performed effort-
lessly and indefatiguably. Perceptual variations can also modulate fatigue. If work output is perceived as being insignificant or inappropriate, fatigue onset is accelerated.

Finally, an important modifier of energy reserves is success or
satisfaction with the results of the expended effort. Hard, gruel-
ing work which leads to satisfying results, success and a sense of
accomplishment seems to unlock reserves of energy that attenu-
ate fatigue; fruitless labor seems to lower the threshold for weariness. This psychological divergence is a very powerful one and
will prove to be an important cog in the endeavor to tame fatigue.

Excessive natural fatigue is easy to predict. Any activity that
leads to energy depletion or any work that leads to unsatisfactory
results will induce it. Overwork, over-exercise, excessive psychological stress, excessive physical stress (such as very hot and hu-
mid environments, noise pollution), synchronization stress (shift

work, jet-lag) and insufficient rest will lead to energy depletion. Fruitless work and failure will exacerbate it.

CAUSES OF UNNATURAL FATIGUE

There are innumerable causes of unnatural fatigue. The main categories include:
♦ a serious pathological state of any organ in the body
♦ malfunction of the operational machinery of any organ
♦ psychological dysfunction or psychiatric conditions
♦ insufficient rest as a result of sleep abnormalities
♦ miscellaneous: chronic fatigue syndrome

ORGAN PATHOLOGY AND FATIGUE

A pathological onslaught of any type (degenerative, infiltrative, toxic, cancerous, inflammatory) on any major organ of the body can result in serious incapacitating fatigue. This review is not meant to convert the reader into an instant physician but to impress upon him the incredible variety of afflictions than can underlie a simple symptom such as fatigue. It will also serve as a motivator to seek medical help when indicated and a convenient check-list of conditions to rule out either by clinical examination or by laboratory testing.

Brain:
Several conditions notably Parkinson's disease, multiple sclerosis and several dementias can lead to chronic fatigue; strokes by virtue of rendering physical mobility extremely inefficient and the attendant psychological frustration can be an important source of tiredness. What is characteristic of central nervous system diseases is that they rarely cause fatigue as a sole manifestation. Their presence is usually signaled by a rich array of other overt signs and symptoms (i.e. paralysis).

Heart:

Many conditions of the heart and circulation can produce fatigue and very often as the sole manifestation. Painless heart attacks in the elderly can be perceived as tiredness exclusively. Congestive heart failure can diminish cardiac output and reduce the delivery of oxygen and nutrients to serve the energy needs of the body. Shortness of breath on exertion or swelling of the lower parts of the legs are common signs of this condition. Too slow a heart rate (complete heart block) or too rapid a heart rate (atrial fibrillation) can also lead to a decreased cardiac output and, consequently, fatigue. Fainting spells or dizzy spells, shortness of breath and extremes of pulse rate should lead to an urgent medical evaluation.

Lungs:

Individuals with chronic obstructive lung disease (chronic bronchitis, emphysema) and uncontrolled asthma breathe through a high resistance obstructed bronchial tree. It is almost the equivalent of breathing through a straw 24 hours a day. The excessive work of breathing can lead to rapid energy depletion. Several other lung diseases (diffuse fibrosis, blood clots) not only lead to a chronic respiratory muscle overload but also lead to hypoxia (reduced oxygen in the blood because of abnormal gas exchange) which will obviously aggravate the sense of fatigue. The cardinal symptoms of these diseases are shortness of breath and coughing.

Gastro-intestinal tract:

Any intestinal pathology that interferes with the absorption of food will result in a state of malnutrition and cachexia (end-result of starvation). Inflammatory bowel disease (Ulcerative colitis, Crohn's disease) can lead to a debilitated state. Most important, however, is the potential for gastro-intestinal blood leakage to result in severe blood loss or iron-deficiency anemia. This is a very important cause of fatigue because of its prevalence and medical gravity. Cancers of the grastro-intestinal tract frequently present this way. One should be wary of abdominal pains, new diarrhea or constipation and especially a drastic change in the color of the stools (too pale suggests malabsorption, too dark, blood

loss).
Liver:
Chronic hepatitis such as hepatitis B and C (blood transfusions) or advanced cirrhosis of the liver (alcohol) are often associated with chronic fatigue. Any individual with chronic fatigue who has ever received a transfusion of blood should be thoroughly screened.
Pancreas:
Digestive enzymes and insulin (diabetes mellitus) are key products of this unglamorous organ. Maldigestion will lead to malnutrition which will, in turn, lead to enfeeblement. Decompensated diabetes mellitus leads to severe dehydration, profound metabolic and electrolytic disturbances and, almost regularly, fatigue. Diabetes mellitus may be insidious in onset and will often signal its presence by causing excessive urination and thirst.
Biliary tract:
Chronic obstruction causes metabolic disturbances and leads to the absence of biliary contents to assist digestion (leads to maldigestion).
Endocrine:
Glandular dysfunction, resulting in either too little or excessive production of hormones, cause severe fatigue. Hyperthyroidism (excess of thyroid hormone) accelerates all metabolic processes and leads to a state of energy depletion. Hypothyroidism (insufficient thyroid hormone) is typically associated with languor, sluggishness and inactivity. These two conditions are very important conditions to rule out medically when confronted with a problem of unexplained chronic fatigue. Hypoadrenalism (decreased adrenal gland hormones) and hypopituitarism (diminished hormone production from the pitutary gland) are other notable examples. Testosterone deficiency is probably a significant contributor to fatigue in the ageing male. Special emphasis should be placed on thyroid gland dysfunction. Excessive or insufficient thyroid hormones are an exceedingly important cause of unexplained fatigue and not at all uncommon. In fact, a thyroid profile or screen is almost routine in general medical practice simply because the con-

ditions are insidious and difficult to diagnose clinically. Signs and symptoms that one should be on the look-out for:

♦ Excessive thyroid hormone (hyperthyroidism)
- feeling "hot" all the time (heat intolerance)
- nervousness
- emotional lability
- insomnia
- tremulousness
- diarrhea
- excessive sweating
- excellent appetite
- weight loss
- muscular weakness
- rapid heart beat, palpitations
- retracted eye lids or a stare
- eyes bulging out
- thinning of hair and skin
♦ Insufficient thyroid hormone (hypothyroidism)
- fatigue
- lethargy
- constipation
- intolerance to cold
- muscular cramps
- heavy menses
- loss of appetite
- slowness of movements
- raucous voice
- swelling of eyelids
- thickened tongue
- general puffiness of face
- cold skin
- tough skin
- diminished reflexes

The presence of these signs and symptoms is a clear indication

for screening tests.
Haematologic:
Low blood count or anemia is a prime cause of fatigue. Its presence demands extensive medical investigation because there are literally hundreds of different disease processes that can cause anemia. Leukemias (cancer of white blood cells) are profoundly debilitating.
Kidneys:
Chronic renal failure from any cause is associated with diminished vigor to downright torpor. Its detection depends on blood tests. Certain conditions of the kidneys cause dehydration or imbalances in the mineral content of the blood (sodium and potassium among others) that can lead not only to fatigue but to a complete state of muscular paralysis. Severe fatigue is a hallmark symptom of renal failure. The diagnosis depends on a simple biochemical determination on a blood sample.
Muscle:
Diffuse diseases of muscle (myositis, dystrophies) lead to weakness and secondarily to fatigue. An intriguing condition called Myasthemia Gravis (dysfunction of the neuromuscular interface due to an attack by antibodies) needs specific testing to rule out. The critical clue to this illness is the presence of actual muscular weakness, which is generally not the case with global fatigue.
Bones:
A condition called Paget's disease is due to an overbundance of bone production whose intrinsic blood supply so expands the circulation that it can cause what is called high-output congestive heart failure. The fatigue is secondary to the congestive heart failure.
Skin:
Diffuse inflammatory diseases of the skin can also lead to high-output congestive heart failure (by expanding the circulation and causing volume overload). In addition to this, heavy desquamation can cause protein deficiency and the chronic discomfort, energy depletion.

Systemic pathology:
This refers to diseases that are not organ specific but diffuse in their effect. Disseminated cancer is self-explanatory. Unfortunately, disseminated cancer is so lethal that the presence of asthenia is hardly the dominant issue. Chronic infections are an extremely important category of illness in the realm of unnatural protracted fatigue. Generally, this clinical state of fatigue and debility occurs with generalized infections (as opposed to localized). Bacterial and fungal infections feature most prominently tuberculosis and bacterial endocarditis (an infection localized on a heart valve with continuous seeding of the general circulation). Bacterial endocarditis not infrequently manifests itself as a progressive asthenic state and, in the absence of additional overt signs and symptoms can be easily missed. It takes a very thorough and astute physician to "pick up" this illness in its early stages. The same comments can be made for tuberculosis. This is an eminently "missable" illness and should always be considered in the differential diagnosis of unexplained fatigue. A negative PPD test and a normal chest X-ray rules it out for practical purposes. Endocarditis can be ruled out with blood cultures although there are many exceptions to this rule.

Viral infections distinguish themselves in the group of illnesses most likely to feature fatigue prominently. In this group there are:

- HIV causing AIDS
- hepatitis B and C
- infectious mononucleosis
- Lyme disease
- post-viral asthenia, which is a prolonged state of fatigue following an acute viral infection (almost any virus)

Fortunately the first three viral syndromes are easily diagnosed with specific laboratory tests. Any thoughtful physician would perform them if the index of suspicion is high.

Parasitic infestation, as a cause of chronic fatigue, is not an important consideration in North America, but in the economically-deprived tropical areas of the world, they should be specifically ruled out with the appropriate diagnostic work-up.

METABOLIC DYSFUNCTION OF ORGANS

The engines of organ function, the biochemical machinery of metabolic processes will cause significant fatigue when malfunctioning. A deficiency of fuel or nutrients deprives the metabolic processes of the necessary energy to fulfill their duties: a deficiency of oxygen (hypoxia, anemia, carboxyhemoglobinemia and methemoglobinemia) or an insufficiency in the delivery of oxygen because of vascular disease (obstruction, fistulas); deficiencies in essential nutrients (sugars, proteins, fats), vitamins and minerals. The medical conditions that lead to these deficiencies have to be systematically rooted out: malnutrition, malabsorption, anorexia and bulimia nervosa, wasting of proteins either through the gastrointestinal or renal tracts.

The biochemical machinery can also malfunction for a myriad of other reasons: enzyme deficiencies either acquired or congenital (enzymes are accelerators of chemical reactions), toxicities of all types, drug side-effects, radiation damage and chronic overwork such as excessive exercise.

Two of the above stand out as fatigue-inducing champions: drugs and toxic substances. Drug side-effects are an exceedingly important potential cause of fatigue. Physicians are always alert to this possibility when prescribing medications. When a particular medication is suspected of being the culprit, a simple cessation and re-challenge procedure usually settles the issue (there is no specific test to detect a drug side-effect such as fatigue). Many classes of pharmaceuticals can induce fatigue. Beta-blockers used to treat hypertension and heart disease are probably the most frequent offenders. Almost all antihypertensives, sedatives, cholesterol-lowering drugs, and the list could go on and on, will at one time or another, quite unpredictably induce a state of fatigue. The main point here is to always suspect a pharmaceutical drug as potentially responsible for the problem. Non-pharmaceutical drugs

such as alcohol, nicotine and "hard" drugs are likewise possible pros-
trating agents. Very few people realize that cigarette smoking in and of
itself is a serious pilferer of energy stores. Alcohol excess and cigarette smoking can convert an energetic go-getter into a torpid slouch.

We are literally immersed in a sea of environmental or industrial
toxic substances. Slow, insidious intoxication is occasionally a cause
of chronic fatigue. The total environment, nature, home or work place
should be scrutinized for any offending agent. From pesticides and
herbicides to carbon monoxide, various dusts and home-use solvents,
there is a bewildering array of potential intoxications that one must
systematically rule out in the appropriate setting. For example, chronic
fatigue in a car mechanic working in a poorly-ventilated garage could
be the result of carbon monoxide poisoning. The same would apply to
someone living just above the indoor parking of an apartment building. Any industrial exposure (be it liquid, fumes or dust) should be
suspected until proven innocent.

A related syndrome, the so called Sick Building Syndrome, is a
significant consideration. Sick-building syndrome refers to a constellation of symptoms, principally fatigue, malaise, headaches and irritation of mucous membranes that have been traced back to the air quality of sealed buildings with centrally controlled mechanical ventilation.
This syndrome surfaced in the 1970s when the overall ventilation of
buildings was reduced to conserve energy. The probable cause of this
condition is an inadequate dilution of irritants arising from building
materials (formaldehyde and others), developer's solutions and personal care products. The treatment revolves around improving ventilation.

Multiple-chemical sensitivity is another slippery syndrome that
is difficult to prove. Some people develop a variety of symptoms
such as fatigue, malaise, headaches and dizziness when exposed
to low levels of commonly encountered chemicals. From perfumes
to exhaust fumes, paints and solvents, they seem to be exquisitely
sensitive to them and become ill or incapacitated. Because there
is no diagnostic test for this condition, a high index of suspicion is
required to establish it as a cause of chronic fatigue. The only known

treatment is avoidance of exposure.

PSYCHOLOGICAL DYSFUNCTION AS A CAUSE OF FATIGUE

Depression, neuroses and psychoses are not infrequently associated with fatigue. Depression is the most important. It might well be one of the most frequent causes of unrelenting fatigue. What complicates the picture is the difficulty in making a diagnosis. Depression can be subtle, insidious, and episodic and can masquerade as a physical ailment. This diagnosis should always be entertained particularly if all physical causes have been ruled out. Mild depression can be easily overlooked by yourself and your physician.

Neuroses are often the root cause of fatigue. It is not the "neurological work" of aberrant psychology that is responsible but the systemic neuro-hormonal activation triggered by anxiety or worry and the inefficiency of daily living that depletes energy stores (i.e. fidgeting).

Psychoses, by their very graveness are usually fairly obvious and appropriate therapy becomes a befitting undertaking for a professional in the field.

Excessive emotional distress will wear out even the most sturdy amongst us. Excessive worry, anxiety, fear, love, hate, joy, suffering, craving, libido, drive, will debilitate a perfectly healthy individual. The explanation is three-fold. There is energy over-consumption (stress hormones such as adrenaline and corticosteroids, activation of the autonomic nervous system, cardiac and respiratory over-stimulation, circulatory hypertension and enhanced heat loss requirement, all lead to metabolic over-work) as well as insufficient rest. Sleep perturbation is almost always part and parcel of emotional distress thus robbing the victim of the restorative qualities of a sound sleep. Inefficient living or pointless activity completes the picture of a severe imbalance in total body energy budgeting. One can simply not underestimate the impact of emotional distress as a cause of disabling fatigue.

A condition commonly referred to as "nervousness" embodies many of the key features of the above psychological dysfunctions. We readily recognize nervous people. They are "hyper,"constantly fidgeting, streaking from one location to another, are frequently tremulous, worry about everything and are super-sensitive to stressful events. They are hyper-reactive and hyper-active. The end-result is severe fatigue: they are "wound-up" psychologically with the attendant constant stimulation of the sympathetic nervous system and stress hormones which lead to an accelerated metabolism and an inefficient lifestyle. They become energy-depleted and, consequently, exhausted.

The psycho-physiological basis of "nervousness" is not known but it seems to be largely an inherited temperamental trait. It thus makes it a difficult entity to modify.

INSUFFICIENT REST

Two thirds of our lives is spent burning calories and the other third, recuperating. A full eight hours of sleep is a biological imperative. No living creature can bypass this mandatory restorative undertaking. The first question a physician will ask a patient complaining of constant tiredness is the status of his sleep both in terms of quantity and quality. For most driven workaholics, sleep is an evil inconvenience. Unfortunately, this mandatory respite is an unforgiving paramour. Issues relating to the quantity of sleep are straightforward. Most people require approximately eight hours of sleep per day. Sleep requirements can vary between six and ten hours per day and each individual spontaneously recognizes his own. That only leaves the wisdom to respect them (sleep requirements).

The real sleeper in this area (pardon the pun) is abnormalities in the quality of sleep. Poor sleep quality is a common cause of chronic fatigue. A famous syndrome, the Pickwickian syndrome, will serve to illustrate the problem. This syndrome portrays an obese, plethoric middle-aged male forever nodding off to sleep in the daytime only to be interrupted by a loud grunting snore. He suffers from respiratory failure and has a much-reduced life expectancy for a number of medical reasons. Reason? Sleep-apnea, causing inadequate depth and duration of restorative sleep. This insufficiency of sleep leads to daytime fatigue, drowsiness and an overwhelming compulsion to doze off, sometimes at the most inopportune time.

Sleep-apnea is a condition that frequently goes unrecognized for decades because the victim is not aware of his dilemma. The sleep mate, however, is made painfully aware of its manifestations. The sleep-apnea victim almost always snores heavily, has periods of non-breathing (no air flow through the mouth) in spite of efforts to breath and these spells of apnea are terminated by a partial arousal associated with a loud grunting gasp as he finally manages to move air. The mechanics are well understood. During deep sleep, pharyngeal muscles relax, collapse and cause upper airway obstruction. Absence of air flow leads to unventilated lungs, therefore no oxygen diffusion into blood, therefore cerebral hypoxia. This state of insufficient oxygen delivery to the brain triggers an arousal reflex which foreshortens phase IV sleep which is qualitatively the most important for restorative purposes. Following hundreds of cycles of apnea, arousal and short-changing of deep sleep in a single night, there emerges a condition of sleep deprivation and chronic fatigue (amongst many other clinically important consequences). Sleep-apnea should be suspected when there is intense snoring and periods of apnea. A definitive diagnosis can be made in the laboratory with specific sleep studies. Because treatment is available, it is a shame to miss this condition in the differential diagnosis of chronic fatigue.

CHRONIC FATIGUE SYNDROME

Special mention of this syndrome is warranted because of the controversies surrounding its very existence and its popularity in the media.

The criteria for the diagnosis of chronic fatigue syndrome are:
- ♦ unexplained, persistent, incapacitating fatigue of new onset
- ♦ plus four or more of the following:
  - impairment of memory and concentration
  - sore throat
  - tender cervical or axillary nodes
  - muscle pains
  - multi-joint pain without inflammation
  - headaches of a new pattern
  - un-refreshing sleep
  - post-exertional malaise lasting ~ 24 hours

The core of this illness is unbearable exhaustion. A very frequent accompanying symptom is depression (two thirds).

The etiology of this syndrome is up in the air. One school of thought favors an infectious causation based on a myriad of inconsistent findings: frequently follows a flu-like illness, viral antibodies against several viruses have been detected, immunologic abnormalities can be detected plus a variety of other esoteric findings. Because depression is a frequent accompaniment and because emotional stress exacerbates the symptoms, a second school of thought suggests that the syndrome is fundamentally psychiatric. The battle lines are delineated. Is the syndrome a physical ailment with reactive psychological disturbances or vice-versa?

This illness presents an exceptional challenge to the treating physician. He is dealing with an individual profoundly incapacitated by unrelenting exhaustion with no diagnostic test to confirm a diagnosis, no specific therapy and the exasperating unspoken hypothesis that the whole problem might be psychological. This dilemma makes dealing with hypochondriasis seem like child's play.

A lot of fuss is made about this syndrome. My personal feeling is that it is a mixed bag of conditions of varied etiologies all sharing a common denominator of severe disabling fatigue. A specific label may afford a psychological crutch but it has no other practical value. In the absence of specific therapy, there is not much to gain by playing a labeling game. The approach or strategies are the same as would apply to any victim of chronic fatigue without a specific reversible cause.

CHAPTER 5
AN APPROACH TO PROBLEM FATIGUE

The first step is to determine if a problem actually exists or not. Because fatigue is largely subjective, at least in its early stages and milder forms, only you can decide if there is a point at issue. This decision is generally based on past experience. New-onset fatigue clearly departing from a previous pattern should ring alarm bells. Any fatigue which is severe, not obviously explained by common sense logic and which interferes with every-day living or enjoyment of life, should be looked into. If, in your judgment, there is "something wrong", then your intuition is probably right. There can be something wrong.

The second step is to establish if the abnormal state of fatigue is likely to be natural or pathological. Table 4.1 in Chapter 4 lists some of the characteristics that help in differentiating them. When in doubt, assume that the fatigue is unnatural until proven otherwise.

Table 5.1 summarizes the different steps in dissecting the problem and elaborating a provisional diagnosis that will orient the therapeutic approach.

Natural fatigue is a mild, non-incapacitating inner sensation of weariness usually proportionate to the inciting conditions. The fundamental fatigue-producing state is a disequilibrium between work demand, work capacity and the sufficiency of rest. While one would assume that common sense would prevail here, and that each and every one of us would have a fairly accurate grasp of what our personal equilibrium is, this is not always the case. Denial, distorted perceptions, mindlessness, blind obstinacy are but a few of the many de-railers of common sense. When in doubt about the genesis of problem fatigue, one might want to consult an objective third party to obtain an honest opinion. For most people, a friend, spouse, sibling, parent or family physician will settle the issue.

If it is resolved that a straightforward dysequilibrium in sup-ply-demand is responsible for the exacerbated state of fatigue then its management is utterly transparent.

Unnatural fatigue is suffocating and the more so because, at the outset, it often is inexplicable. It is a clear break from past experience, it is disabling, very unpleasant, lasts all day and simply does not respond to increased rest. The victim senses that there is something "very wrong" going on. Can a well-informed individual sort it out on his own? Probably. While this might be the most economical way to solve the mystery, it might not be the most prudent. There is everything to gain and nothing to lose by systematically excluding important conditions, especially medical and psychological ones. It is quite tragic to miss perfectly treat-able illnesses out of either laziness or recklessness.

TABLE 5.1
DECISIONAL TREE OF PROBLEM FATIGUE

DETERMINE SIGNIFICANCE
OF FATIGUE

Natural Fatigue   Unnatural Fatigue

Evaluate   Rule Out a
Disequilibrium   Medical Condition

Rule Out A Psychological
Dysfunction

Assess For:
Stress Overload
Emotional Overload

Assess Lifestyle Issues

Assess Basics:
Nutrition
Sleep/Rest
Physical Conditioning

Significant Fatigue of
Unknown Cause

RULE OUT A MEDICAL CONDITION

Used in its broadest sense, a medical condition includes a wide array of illnesses either internally or externally-generated. The sheer breadth and complexity of the field makes it mandatory that a physician take charge. The following action plan is recommended:

- Consult a family physician or a general internist.
- Make that visit fully dedicated to the issue of fatigue.
- Impress on your physician that this problem is real and that you are very worried about it. Explain your rationale for believing that this problem is significant (you want to break through the usual skepticism that builds up in a physician's mind after years of dealing with neurotic or hypochondriacal patients).
- Prepare your description of the symptoms ahead of time and know the answers to the typical questions that a physician will ask: since when, how severe, the pattern, what activities aggravate or alleviate the symptoms, associated symptoms, all known current or past medical problems, all medications consumed, a brief description of your work and work place, nutritional, sleep and exercise habits. When well prepared, you can crystallize the constellation of information that is invaluable to your doctor. Of course, he will have more pointed questions depending on his suspicions.
- Once the clinical evaluation is completed, indicate to your doctor (unless done as a matter of fact) that routine or screening laboratory tests would be of great help in reassuring you and that for your peace of mind, they should be done (in this world of hidden incentives and disincentives, it is not always clear when and why laboratory tests are done or not).
- Assuming that a clinical diagnosis is not in the offing, the following screening tests are perfectly reasonable:
   - complete blood count
   - renal function (BUN, Creatinine) and electrolytes, urinalysis
   - liver functions (enzymes, bilirubin)

- serum proteins
- sedimentation rate
- thyroid profile
- chest X-ray
- ECG

When a specific disease is thought responsible, consultation with the appropriate specialist and relevant investigative testing is expected.

In the case of a suspected industrial poison or a domestic intoxicant, special investigative efforts must be focused on the situation at hand. The possibilities here are endless.

As already discussed, if a pharmaceutical agent (i.e. beta-blockers) is surmised, a trial of cessation and rechallenge might be done to eliminate all doubt.

RULE OUT A PSYCHOLOGICAL DYSFUNCTION

The two foremost malefactors are depression and chronic anxiety neurosis. The former because of its prevalence, insidiousness and eminent treatability; the latter will not only sap you of all your discretionary energy supplies but it will literally torture you with psychic pain. Both are scourges of the human condition and should be systematically excluded.

Depression is such a common human experience that it may be difficult to differentiate normal everyday reactive depression and a pathological state.

The key is to have a sense of what is habitual for a person and what is out of the ordinary. As with any other aspect of human nature, there is a built-in genetically programmed emotional setpoint around which we oscillate throughout our lives. Some people are naturally inclined to melancholy and others tend to be rather upbeat, simply on a temperamental basis. The standard against which one will apply the diagnostic criteria will vary from individual to individual. This is why a reference to a person's habitual mood on a life-long basis is critical.

The symptoms or features that one should look for to ferret out a diagnosis of depression are:

- Five (or more) of the following symptoms have been present during two weeks (or more):
1. Depressed mood most of the day
2. Markedly diminished interest or pleasure in almost all activities most of the day
3. Significant weight loss or weight gain or decrease or increase in appetite nearly every day.
4. Insomnia or excessive sleep nearly every day.
5. Psychomotor agitation or retardation (hyperactive or hypoactive).
6. Fatigue or loss of energy nearly every day.
7. Feelings of worthlessness or excessive or inappropriate guilt every day.
8. Diminished ability to think or concentrate or indecisiveness nearly every day.
9. Recurrent thoughts of death or suicide.
- The symptoms cause clinically significant distress or impairment in important areas of functioning (social, occupational)
- The symptoms cannot be explained by substance abuse, a medical condition or bereavement.

If a diagnosis of depression seems possible or probable, one should seek professional help not just to confirm the diagnosis but to supervise the whole course of therapy. Long term follow-up is essential for optimal results. Your family doctor, psychologist or psychiatrist, either individually or concurrently, will guide you through the minefield of depression.

Chronic anxiety neurosis is the second prominent psychological cause of fatigue. This should not be surprising because constant worry and nervousness activate a host of physiologic "protective" mechanisms to maintain homeostasis. Almost every system in the body participates. From the central nervous system flows torrents of nervous stimulation (sympathetic nervous sys-

tem) and neuroendocrine release (trophic hormones from the hypo-
thalamus and pituitary gland). The physiologic responses include increases in physical activity (trembling, fidgetiness, tenseness, accelerated pace), an increase in blood pressure (constriction of the vascular
bed), in heart rate, in respiratory rate, in metabolic rate and metabolic
inefficiencies (effect of catecholamines and corticosteroids). All these
effects, plus more, exact a heavy price in energy expenditure. If you
couple this with the almost inevitable presence of poor sleep performance, one can see how the prerequisites for fatigue are all in place.

An anxiety neurosis, like depression, has a large grey zone where it
is not clear what should be considered normal or abnormal. Like depression, a thoughtful reference to past experience might be helpful.
Ultimately, each individual must analyze their own circumstances and
decide. The following list of diagnostic criteria for an anxiety neurosis
might be of assistance:

- Excessive anxiety and worry lasting for a majority of days
  of six months duration about a number of events or activities.
- The person finds it difficult to control the worry.
- The worry and anxiety are associated with three or more of
  the following six symptoms: (1) restlessness, keyed up,
  on edge, (2) easy fatiguability, (3) difficulty concentrating
  or mind going blank, (4) irritability, (5) muscle tension,
  (6) sleep disturbance.
- The worry, anxiety or physical symptoms cause clinically
  significant distress or impairment in social, occupational
  or other important areas of functioning.
- The disturbance is not due to the effects of drug abuse, a
  medication or a general medical condition, does not occur
  exclusively during a mood disorder, psychotic disorder or
  a pervasive developmental disorder.
- The focus of the anxiety and worry is not confined to but
  may be allied to panic attacks, social phobias, obsessive-
  compulsive disorder, separation anxiety, gaining weight,
  hypochondriasis and do not occur exclusively during a

postraumatic stress disorder.

These criteria are gleaned from the diagnostic and statistical manual of mental disorders of the American Psychiatric Association. The distinction between a generalized anxiety disorder and "normal" anxiety is dependent on the proper weighting of "excessive" and "difficult to control" and on the presence or absence of significant impairment or distress. This distinction is highly subjective.

Any suspicion that an anxiety neurosis is instrumental in your predicament should lead to professional consultation. Starting point - your family doctor.

EXAMINE YOUR LIFE FOR THE PRESENCE OF STRESS OR EMOTIONAL OVERLOAD

Are you being whiplashed by the furious frenzy of stressful entanglements? Are you emotionally bled dry? These are extremely efficient wasters of energy and will leave you as limp as a wet rag given the right circumstances. Most of us will have either experienced a major stressful event or have witnessed it to see the connection. Observe somebody going through a divorce, death of a loved one, a legal suit, loss of a job, sudden illness etc. See how energetic they are!

The draining effects of stress are not only operative with major stressful events, but the same result takes place with the cumulative effect of much smaller but more numerous stressful occurrences. This is where a misdiagnosis can be made. Innumerable small daily stresses could wear you out and you don't realize it because none of them stand out as being particularly significant. The cumulative effect, though, can demolish you.

One must go through the exercise of objectively analyzing every single aspect of one's life and quantify the stress content. In the event that a careful evaluation does not yield a clear result, the use of a standard validated stress scale might be of assistance. These estimates of stress can give you a rough idea if this factor is weighty in your life. The basic structure is as follows: there is a series of questions on your assessment of how you feel about and how you respond to an array of life situations. The answers are given a rating number. After adding up the rating numbers, one concludes with a score that indicates the probability that stress is minor or major. This can be a useful guide. Because these questionnaires tend to be long, no attempt will be made to reproduce them here.. Furthermore, different stress scales have been devised for different circumstances, i.e. professional stress, marital stress, non-specific psychological stress and so on. This information is easily found in your library or on the internet.

Emotional overload is a virtual ally of stress. It is simple to recognize. Excessive grief, hate, love, craving, joy, all positive or negative emotions in their extreme will wear you out as surely as running a marathon. A casual assessment of one's daily preoccupations and feelings will make the diagnosis evident. The difficulty with emotional overload does not lie in the diagnosis but in the remedy.

EVALUATE YOUR LIFESTYLE

You can run on the fast track or the slow one. If you choose the fast track, you better be qualified or proficient to handle it. It is not a matter of loving it or hating it, it is a matter of just simple "too much". Too much of anything. Your machinery is built to run at a cruising rate of 3,000 r.p.m. If you insist on operating at 5,000 r.p.m. on a sustained basis, you will burn up and burn out. A chronic state of fatigue will set in. As it should. It is there to protect you against burning up.

Common sense should prevail here. If you get up at 5:30 a.m. to rush to the gym and play one hour of racquetball before work, then consume a 2,000 calorie fat-laden breakfast, work 10 hours straight skipping lunch (you feel guilty about breakfast), drink 12 cups of coffee during your frenzied 10 hours of innovative and revolutionary work, be the assigned entertainer of your work mates, rush to night school 2 nights per week, juggle a couple of girlfriends on alternate evenings (you just can't decide which one you love most), drink alcohol more than you should, secretly consume your 8 cigarettes per day that you just can't give up, wolf down a 16 oz steak for supper in record time and simply will not go to sleep until you have flicked your TV to death, and then, while trying to fall asleep, you ruminate about the racquetball tournament awaiting you on the weekend wondering when you will fit in all the studying that has already backlogged, of course you'll be tired! Wouldn't we all be?

EVALUATE HOW YOU MANAGE THE BASICS OF HEALTHY LIVING

The basics of healthy living in the context of fatigue prevention are nutrition, sleep and physical conditioning. All three must be assessed for their appropriateness both quantitatively and qualitatively. If you have insufficient personal knowledge to make a valid judgment, then either inform yourself or seek the enlightenment of a professional. Neglect in this area, particularly poor sleep habits, can wreck an otherwise wholesome way of life.

My personal opinion is that for most people who complain of fatigue, the problem can be traced back to a lack of thoughtful adherence to the basic rules of healthy living. Obesity, chronic sleep deprivation, poor physical conditioning and inadequate stress management largely underlie the bulk of life-limiting fatigue.

There is a simple test to determine the extent to which any of the basics are contributing to a lack of resistance to fatigue. Trial and error. The contrast of enhanced vigor after correcting a deficiency, be it sleep by sleeping more or physical conditioning after an inspired training program would be proof enough that there was a problem in those areas (retrospectively). In any event, the trial is a gain-gain endeavour.

WHEN NO EXPLANATION CAN BE FOUND

At the end of the diagnostic process as delineated in the decisional tree of problem fatigue, one may conclude that there is no satisfactory explanation for the state of protracted fatigue. In medicine, we cover up this embarrassing mystery with the learned esoteric term "idiopathic". Our textbooks of medicine are riddled with the term "idiopathic". It translates into "we simply do not know."

If you suffer from idiopathic fatigue, the options available for treatment are reduced. After deeper investigations (generally not that productive) and repeated investigations (occasionally abnormal laboratory results only appear later in the course of an illness) one may have to conclude that the condition has no detectable etiology. Nevertheless, periodic re-evaluations are a wise investment both for late detection of a fastidious medical problem and for fine-tuning of any therapeutic strategy.

CHAPTER 6
THE TREATMENT OF CHRONIC FATIGUE

This is the heart of the matter. The mission of this expose is to palliate or cure unrelenting fatigue and rediscover a happy and productive life. Why short-change yourself? If you feel excessive fatigue is dampening your gusto for life there are certainly valuable tools for you in the upcoming chapters. If you delude yourself into thinking that you can simply do battle with fatigue, defy it with complete disregard for its incontrovertible biological role, you are in for serious grief. Unheeded fatigue is harmful.

There is another person who is targeted by this book. He is epitomized by your all-American Paladin who pushes himself to accumulate even more almighty bucks, experiencing fatigue regularly and substantially, and seemingly coping well, oblivious to the subtle nefariousness of his moderate free-floating fatigue. What a shame! To miss out on the treasures of maximum vitality and the exhilaration of high-energy dynamism. There is no reason to impose a tax on your life's venture out of sheer neglect.

The therapeutic strategies developed in this book parallel in a certain way the diagnostic decisional tree in Table 5.1

- Apply specific therapy to a causative medical (physical or mental) affliction.
- Management of stress and emotional overload.
- Adjustment of lifestyle excesses or aberrations.
- Strengthen the foundations of health maintenance.
- The non-specific treatment of idiopathic fatigue.
- Pharmacological therapy.
- Natural and alternative medicines: fact or fiction.

CHAPTER 7
WHEN THE CAUSE OF FATIGUE
IS A PHYSICAL OR MENTAL ILLNESS

The discovery of a physical illness as the root cause of chronic fatigue is paradoxically a godsend. It is so, because in most instances, effective therapy is available. Perfect scenario. Find an illness, cure it and case closed. Though chronic fatigue is not often the result of a clear-cut medical problem, the first step is to rule it out.

PHYSICAL ILLNESS

Several examples will serve to illustrate the benefits of good medical care.

In hormonal deficiency states such as hypothyroidism (low thyroid hormone production), or Addison's disease (low corticosteroid production), simple hormonal replacement therapy is, for practical purposes, curative. Overnight, one can be transformed from a debilitated invalid to a bouncy dynamo. Hyperthyroidism (excessive thyroid hormone production) which will burn you to the ground, can be controlled with surgery, radiotherapy or anti-thyroid drugs. Sex hormone deficiencies, particularly testosterone in the male, may well shore up the sagging energies of the ageing male but this is, as yet, the be clearly demonstrated in appropriate studies. Uncontrolled diabetes mellitus is easily rectified. Tight blood sugar control with insulin is a boon for a sense of well-being.

I have seen in my practice countless cases of incessant fatigue caused by abnormal heart rhythms. Instances where the heart rate is too slow (sick sinus syndrome, complete electrical heart block) will be "cured" with the installation of a permanent pacemaker. When the heart beat is too rapid (tachycardias, atrial fibrillation), judicious anti-arrhythmic therapy is of tremendous benefit. Congestive heart failure, which is becoming a medical problem of ever-increasing prevalence in our society, is substantially improved with well-devised drug therapy.

Infectious diseases of all kinds, be they indolent, localized or systemic, are totally eradicable with powerful modern antibiotics. Even viral illnesses, against which until very recently the medical profession was helpless, will now yield to anti-viral medications. There is, as yet, no true eradicating treatment for viral diseases (note HIV and hepatitis B, C) but certain aspects of the clinical manifestations will improve considerably with modern drugs.

Chronic renal failure will yield to dialysis, poor asthma control to good bronchodilator therapy, chronic non-infectious systemic inflammatory disorders (systemic lupus erythematosus) to immuno-suppressive therapy and several cancers to chemotherapy or radiotherapy. The list is endless. The key is to detect the illness and then leave the remedy in the hands of an expert.

ENVIRONMENTAL STRESSES AND POISONS

Generally speaking, environmental hazards include anything external to the body that has a negative impact on health, particularly in the context of fatigue. The home and work environment hold a vast array of potential threats to health. When suspected of provoking unnatural fatigue, and this is the critical pivot, they must be unearthed as the actual treatment is unambiguous: you remove or correct the offending agent.

The home environment may be vitiated by overcrowding, poor ventilation, excessive cold, heat dryness, humidity, excessive noise, dust, chemical exposure or poisons: formaldehyde, carbon monoxide, phenolhexachlorophene, sodium hypochlorite (Javex) ammonia (window washing agent, carpet cleaner), sodium and potassium hydroxide (oven cleaner) stain removers, varnishes (turpentine, zylene, toluene, acetone), fluorohydric acid (anti-rust), pesticides (malathion), freon emissions (air conditioning), toxic pigments (paint), pottery (barium, lead, chrome), soldering fumes, glues (organic cyanates etc), photography-developing (silver salts), gardening (insecticides, fungicides, herbicides) swimming pool (chemicals, fungicides), and more.

The opportunities for adverse health consequences are numerous but, in actual fact, it is uncommon for the root cause of fatigue to be traced to the home environment. It only takes a few minutes of reflection to exclude these factors from consideration and the exercise is worthwhile. In some cases, one might find that certain elements of the home environment are contributors to a state of weariness of multi-factorial causation. The correction of these aggravating factors would then become part of a comprehensive program of fatigue management.

The work environment is likewise a possible witch's brew for insidious enfeeblement:

> excessive physical demands
> excessive noise
> visual pollution (computer screen)
> exposure to fumes
> heavy metal poisoning
> exposure to industrial chemicals (30,000 at last count)
> excessive heat, cold, dryness, humidity
> commuting

night shifts
sick building syndrome
multiple-chemical reactivity

Commuting, especially when long, noisy, stressful and unpredictable, is exhausting. When this factor alone dominates the landscape, the solution is obvious.

Night shifts, because of the constant mismatching of physical activities and the hormonal environment tied to the diurnal cycles of day and night (synchronization stress) are debilitating. A worker subjected to changing shifts on a tight, rotating schedule, is a high risk for a state of chronic fatigue. The treatment consists of either eliminating shift work or lengthening the rotation cycles to allow full recovery between changes.

Sick Building Syndrome has already been alluded to. This is a difficult diagnosis to make. Psychological factors muddy the waters. If one determines there are several other individuals in a given building who share the symptoms of SBS, the case is strengthened. The pattern of symptoms is also helpful diagnostically. If fatigue and irritation are consistently associated with working within the building and consistently disappear when out, a probable diagnosis is made. The treatment consists of changing environments or improving ventilation either centrally or locally (by installing unsealed windows).

Multiple-chemical sensitivity also alluded to in a previous chapter is occasionally an issue in the workplace. The problem is proving the relationship between exposure and fatigue. If there exists such a cause-and-effect relationship, avoidance of exposure is the only remedy.

Finally, the outdoors environment contains its own perils. Any extreme in climatic conditions is potentially debilitating. Innumerable exposures (waste site gases, incinerators, contaminated soil, water and plants) should all be systematically excluded when relevant. As with any environmental danger, the essence of management is the detection and correction of the hazard.

PSYCHOLOGICAL ILLNESS

Psychological illnesses are definitely amenable to sensible medical therapy. For the past century, they were treated primarily by psychotherapy (with muted success), but in modern times, there surfaced a veritable explosion in novel pharmacological treatments that have been nothing short of revolutionary. With the onset of the third millennium, nobody needs to remain in the tyrannical clutches of depression or anxiety.

Let it not be misunderstood. Pharmacotherapy has not replaced psychotherapy, it has complemented it. Psychotherapy is still extremely useful for emotional and psychological support.

Pharmacotherapy has really come of age. Its very success has confirmed, to a certain extent, the widespread belief that many psychiatric conditions, primarily major depression and neuroses are truly "hard" organic diseases and not pure emotional aberrations. Depression, for example, is largely a neurotransmitter disease.

Depression and anxiety neuroses are the most closely associated with abnormal fatigue states. Anxiety neuroses will be dealt with in another chapter.

Depression and fatigue are intimately linked and represent a twin burden for the individual and society as a whole. The cost to society is incalculable, let alone the personal devastation that it wreaks. Fatigue is a prominent symptom of depression and is invariably present as a contributor. Depression breeds fatigue and fatigue begets depression.

Depression runs the gamut from a severe paralysis of life's activities to a mild melancholic mood. The former must be treated by a professional and the latter will usually respond to simple measures.

Major depression is essentially an inherited flaw in the brain's biochemistry. If you have a positive family history for a major depression or a bipolar disorder (manic-depressive illness), there is a 30% chance that you will be afflicted with it. This scourge of humanity is still branded as a stigma variably depicted as a character flaw or the result of poor upbringing. Nothing can be further from the truth. Depression is as organic as diabetes and strokes are.

The more severe the depression, the more likely it is genetically-determined (a result of dysfunctional neurochemistry) and the more the sufferer will require top professional help and drug therapy. The therapies available for serious depression:

- ♦ Psychiatric care: if you suffer from a significant depressive illness (significant is when it affects your daily living), you should, as a first step, put yourself under the care of a psychiatrist. He is the best qualified practitioner; after all, he is specifically trained to deal with this illness. Why should you settle for anything less?

- ♦ Psychotherapy: this traditional mode of treatment is still very useful and remains part and parcel of the overall therapeutic approach. Drugs alone will not cure the illness and their effectiveness is variable. Psychotherapeutic support fills in the gaps. The psychiatrist is in a position to choose the most appropriate formula for your specific needs.

- ♦ Anti-depressant drugs: they are the mainstay of modern therapy, particularly the new generation of drugs which have revolutionized the field. The earlier antidepressant drugs, the tricyclic antidepressants (elavil, endep, triavil) have been largely supplanted by the newcomers, the SSRI group of drugs (specific serotonin reuptake inhibitors: Prozac, Zoloft, Luvox, Paxil, Serzone). This gradual shift in choice of drugs was not only fueled by the therapeutic superiority of SSRI's but because of their greater tolerance. Tricyclics are plagued with numerous side-effects, the most frequent being dry mouth, daytime sleepiness, visual disturbances and constipation. SSRI's are certainly not free of side-effects (insomnia and diminished interest in sex) but they are much better tolerated. Not inconsequentially, they are also harder to overdose with; not a detail, when one considers the high suicide risk associated with this disease. Unfortunately, the SSRI's are slow in onset, generally taking three weeks or more to have an effect. This latent period can be cut in half with the addition of another drug (Pindolol).

Pindolol blocks the brain's resistive efforts to the increased flow of serotonin in the synapse. Finally, it is of utmost importance to realize that these drugs, while extremely helpful, do not cure the disease and do not prevent relapses.

♦ Support groups: these self-help groups have become very popular and exist in just about every large and medium-sized metropolitan areas. They provide kinship, education, reassurance, sympathy, reality checks and a sense of purpose.

♦ Electro-convulsive therapy (ECT): given a bad name by the popular media, it is understandably a treatment of last resort. Nevertheless, there is a place for it. It can be life-saving for the most severe forms of depression where the victim is literally imprisoned within a hellish torture chamber that their brain has become for them. The electrical shock alters the brain's electrical and chemical activity and delivers the sufferer from his infernal incarceration.

Mild forms of depression are amenable to self-therapy. "Feeling down," the "blues," melancholy, "in a rut" are all expressions that describe universally experienced temporary lapses in mood. Some more so than others, as there is a strong genetic predisposition to despondency. Glumness and dispiritedness foster and perpetuate fatigue. The lethargy induced by mild depression can be improved to the extent that one is successful in combating the root cause of melancholia. Here follows natural lifters of mood or "blues-busters."

♦ Always looks for a primary cause of "feeling down." So many periods of downheartedness are reactive in nature, reactive to an event such as a loss, failure or bad luck. If you "bust" the cause, you will bust the "blues."

- Always rule out a side-effect from a medication. Sedatives, pain killers, cold medicines and blood pressure medications can all do it. Any drug can, including alcohol. This possibility should be ruled out by stopping and retaking the medication and observing the effects on mood (under supervision of a doctor).

- Act happy and you will be happier. Just as we can put ourselves into a funk by self-induced gloom and doom ideation, we can achieve just the opposite by faking happiness. Act it and you will feel it.

- Avoid isolation: One of the most nefarious aspects of melancholy is that we tend to retreat from close ones and society. That is a mistake. Communing and communicating with someone, especially a friend, spouse, family member, ultimately any one, has an antidepressant effect. Just as depression is contagious, normal mood and toughness are as well. To associate with people, even passively, has a beneficial "drag" effect. In addition to this, the distorted views of life that typically pervade the depressed mind are frequently rectified by simple interaction with a friend.

- Keep busy: The less distracted you are, the more gloom permeates your thoughts. Do anything and keep busy. Get out of the house, go for a long walk, go to a movie, engage in a hobby, work, go shopping, clean the house, wash the dog, shine the car, go to a football game. You name it, you do it. It is a most serious mistake to stop working as a result of mild depression. This is precisely what you should not do. In fact, you should work even more until better times come (and they usually do). Work distracts you and keeps your mental and emotional muscles in good shape.

- List all the things you should be thankful for. You will realize how well off you are, comparatively speaking. If you are not convinced, walk down a medical ward in your local hospital.

♦ Make a reality check: Self-talk is a powerful tool. Talk yourself back to reality. Life is painful. It is an angst-ridden odyssey whose only natural conclusion is death. In this respect we are all equal: we all suffer, we all run a pleasure deficit. We all experience decreased mood at regular intervals, we are all utterly insignificant and no matter how much material we accumulate, no matter how much fame we savor and no matter how much gratification of the flesh we engage in, we are not fundamentally more or less happier than anybody else on earth. Bottom line: get used to it! Look on the bright side. The more depressed you are, the more you will relish the good times when they inevitably come. Think back. Haven't you been melancholic before and eventually snapped out of it?

♦ Do a good deed: Doing something good or generous is a natural mood elevator. There are millions of opportunities in your own back yard to lend a helping hand to somebody. It will make you happier.

♦ Exercise: Exercise is a natural antidepressant. It is very difficult to motivate oneself to exercise when depressed, but if you can muster the inner strength to do it, buoyant dividends will flow. The mechanism of this antidepressant effect is largely unknown. Possibly, the release of endorphins in the brain are, in part, responsible. Whatever the mechanism is, it has been well demonstrated that exercise elevates one's mood and it should be at the core of any strategy to combat mild non-specific depression. *Pari passu,* fatigue relief will follow.

♦ Spiritual healing: Spiritual indulgence is a potent healer of many psychological ills, including depression. The potential benefits are proportionate to the depth and genuineness of the faith. Just rambling off a prayer is of no help whatsoever. It has been indicated in the literature that church-goers have decreased death rates and better over all health. For those inclined, meditation, prayer and soulful bonding with their god might be highly therapeutic.

Seasonal Affective Disorder (SAD), is not, strictly speaking, a psychological illness, but is so closely related to depression that it will be included here. This state of atypical depression exhibits symptoms of fatigue, moodiness, low spirits, loss of motivation and sleep disturbances. It typically occurs in northern climates where the winter is long and harsh and the daylight hours are reduced. People stay indoors for months on end and develop "cabin fever." While the mechanism is unknown, there is a popular theory that the major reason is insufficient sunlight exposure. To the list of "blues-busters" already discussed, one would add a hefty dose of outdoor activities. This gets you out of the house, distracts the mind, refreshes the soul and, if you can "catch some sunshine," so much the better. If the theory about sunlight is correct, there should be some improvement of this mild-winter energy crisis.

CHAPTER 8
WHEN THE ROOT CAUSE IS STRESS OR EMOTIONAL OVERLOAD

Stress is a real or perceived threat to personal security in its broadest sense. What makes an event stressful is a palpable potentiality that harm will come your way physically, psychologically, socially, religiously, professionally, romantically, parentally. The more immediate the danger, the more violent the stress reaction. From the very beginning of evolution, the ability to meet environmental challenges was a prerequisite. Only the successful lineages survived. Part of that successful mix is the appropriate, measured and effective stress reaction.

The most serious threats to a human being are the ones that target his or her fundamental biological missions: to survive, to thrive and to reproduce. Typical stressful events in each category:

Survival
> personal injury or illness
> loss of a job
> retirement

business reorganization
change in financial status
change in career
environmental calamities (earthquake, volcano, major
      storm, electrical blackout)
high-crime neighborhood
committing crimes
unemployment
substance abuse
risky work
being sued
overworked/underworked
heavy mortgage
foreclosure of mortgage or loan
change in responsibilities at work
change in living conditions
jail term
revision of personal habits
change in work hours or conditions
change in residence, school, recreation, church, social ac-
      tivities
time pressures
conflicting beliefs
traveling
transportation
any conflict

Thriving or its perceptual mirror-image, self-esteem
    public speaking
    change in job or financial status
    failing an exam
    failure in a human relationship
    outstanding personal achievement
    spouse begins or stops working
    sexual difficulties

absence of feeling important or significant
physical defects, obesity, disability
any kind of rejection
conflicting values
Reproduction and love
  death of a spouse
  divorce or marital separation/alienation
  death of a close family member
  marriage
  marital reconciliation
  change in health of family member
  death of a friend
  change in number of arguments with spouse
  son or daughter leaving home
  trouble with in-laws
  conflicting loves
  loss of love
  inability to love
The list could go on and on...

The physiological response to a stressful event explains how one can slip into a state of chronic fatigue when overload occurs. There are three components to the stress response: physiological, psychological and behavioral.

The physiological response is designed to protect the organism by arming it for its fight or flight response. This arming mechanism recruits several emergency response systems such as emotional centers, the sympathetic nervous system, the hypothalamic-pituitary-adrenal axis (hormones), the cardiopulmonary system, the metabolic machinery, the immune system and the musculoskeletal apparatus. A typical physiologic response would include fear and worry, release of adrenaline from sympathetic nerve endings and the adrenal medulla, release of corticotropin from the pituitary gland to stimulate the release of cortisol from the adrenal cortex, a sundry of other less important hormones (i.e. to increase blood sugar), an increase in heart rate, blood pressure, strength of cardiac contractions, increase in cardiac output (enhanced oxygen delivery), accelerated respiratory rate, sweating, tensing of muscles, posturing, quickening of all sensory discernments and more. The magnitude of the physiologic stress response tends to mirror the magnitude of the perceived threat.

The psychological response to a stressful event is anxiety. The many facets of anxiety encompass alertness, vigilance, tenseness, uncertainty, a sensation of impending doom, fear, worry and irritation. The mildest form of anxiety is a barely-perceptible sensation of uneasiness but the whole spectrum of the psychological stress reaction extends to the outer limits of terror and panic attacks. These emotional states naturally trigger still more physiological responses in a synergistic way.

Chronic stress can lead to behavioural adjustments in an attempt to mitigate the psychic pain associated with distressing experiences. These compensatory behavioral changes are manifestly necessary for the short-term management of difficult situations but will result in well-entrenched aberrant lifestyles. These stress-induced behavioral defense mechanisms run the gamut from perfectionistic conformity to addictions (attempts to dull psychic pain and anxiety), overwork, crime (best defense is offense) and assorted self-defeating modes of living such as gambling and reclusiveness.

How is stress linked to fatigue? The constellation of physiologic reactions to stress, its psychological repercussions and the compensatory behavioral aberrations that ensue bring about:

- a massive expenditure of energy that exhausts natural energy supplies, which cannot be fully recuperated by rest
- a diminished integrity of the biological machinery itself further exacerbating the equilibrium between energy supply, operating capacity and rest

The latter statement perhaps requires some explanation. Chronic stress not only drains the organism of its available energy supplies but it is directly harmful to cells and organs through a variety of pathological routes. The spectrum runs from vascular atherosclerosis (strokes, heart attacks, renal failure) and cardiac arrhythmias (abnormal beating of the heart) to arthritis, ground out teeth, ulcers, impotence, spastic colon, neuro-dermatitis, diabetes, immune deficiency, accelerated ageing of neurons and a master "aggravator" of any other illness that might have befallen the victim of stress.

The bottom line is this: stress and emotional overload exhaust the organism and create a propitious environment for disease or organ malfunction. Chronic fatigue is the expected result of stress overload. Table 8.1 summarizes the issue.

STRESS MANAGEMENT

Very few amongst us can manipulate the environment to eliminate stressful events, but most of us can improve coping strategies to minimize the impact. There is no magic formula for conquering this scourge of the human condition but there are many steps or benign ruses that will immeasurably improve the quality of our dance with life. Not one stratagem but a confluence of many will help to achieve this goal. There are two fundamental approaches. One is to find ways to minimize exposure to stress and the other is to build up a greater resistance to stress.

KNOW YOURSELF AND ACCEPT YOURSELF

This age-old advice has been a pillar of wisdom since time immemorial. For good reason. Since a lion portion of the stressful content of any experience is a subjective appraisal of the magnitude of the threat and its juxtaposition against the ability of the person to repel that threat, a precise measure of one's capacity, strengths and weaknesses is an essential prerequisite. Otherwise, any mismatch between a false measure of adeptness and reality compounds the danger. If you constantly overestimate your capacity or strength, your stress-driven decisions will expose you to

Table 8.1
STRESS AND FATIGUE

Environmental Challenges   Major Life Events   Trauma, Abuse, Illness

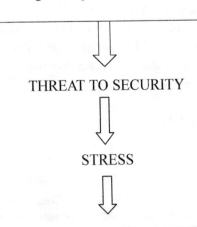

THREAT TO SECURITY

STRESS

ADAPTIVE AND COPING RESPONSES:
PHYSIOLOGICAL: SYMPATHETIC NERVOUS SYSTEM AND STRESS
HORMONES
BEHAVIOURAL: ADAPTIVE AND MALADAPTIVE BEHAVIOUR
PSYCHOLOGICAL: ANXIETY

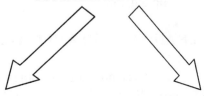

MASSIVE ENERGY EXPENDITURE   OPERATING AND RECUPERATIVE
AND ORGAN DYSFUNCTION   CAPACITY OVERWHELMED

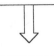

FATIGUE

potential harm. If, on the other hand, you underestimate your capabilities and competence, you will unnecessarily shy away from profitable undertakings. The least vulnerable way to live our lives is to gain a precise, objective and honest knowledge of what our aptitudes are: strengths, weaknesses, temperamental quirks, personality traits, character idiosyncracies, intelligence level, capacity to love, natural resistance to stress, likes and dislikes, stamina, physical and psychological needs, talents and so on. By knowing ourselves accurately, we can navigate the treacherous seas of modern life with a minimum of unwarranted stress. Should a 5'2"-tall teenager invest all his leisure time in perfecting the game of basketball in the hope of someday playing the power forward position on the Chicago Bulls' team? Should a normally obese and naturally plain-looking girl spend all her time and energy training herself to be a runway model? Every pursuit in life must be realistic. It must be based on an intimate knowledge of every facet of the self. This dispassionate cold objectivity is an extremely powerful tool against stress.

Not only should you strive to know yourself well, you must learn to accept yourself and love yourself. Do you really have a choice? No matter how imperfect you are, how dull you are, how homely you are, how anything, you are your only possession for the duration of this journey on earth. You are all you have, you are the only one who truly cares and you are your only source of truth, dignity and destiny. You must love yourself because not doing so is a nonsensical, utterly counterproductive attitude of the mind. If acceptance of yourself does not emerge spontaneously, learn how to do it. How? Gratitude, humility and a deference to the mystery of life.

KNOW YOUR ENVIRONMENT

So many forms of stress are based on irrational fears and exaggerations of dangers borne out of sheer ignorance that the best antidote is knowledge of everything that impacts on your existence. One must acquire a solid knowledge of biology, medicine, sociology, psychology, philosophy, sciences in general, politics etc. The more one knows, the more one understands the inner workings of the living environment, the better one can cope with challenges and, consequently, the less stressful life will be. Don't forget. Stress feeds on ignorance and confusion. Turn on the bright lights of knowledge and dissipate fear.

DISMANTLE BASELESS ANXIETIES

Life is stressful enough not to add to it groundless fears, unreasonable anxieties and unwarranted worrying. Baseless free-floating anxiety is a poison to psychological well-being and a drain of energy stores. Distorted thinking and invalid assumptions about reality continuously trigger false alarms and subject the body to a constant barrage of protective and compensatory physiologic reactions. The long-term effect is toxic and a guarantee of chronic fatigue. Baseless anxieties must be recognized, characterized and dismantled. For most people, simple sensitization to the issues, self-talk and common sense emotional management will suffice. The demolishment of the unknown, which feeds anxiety, and the righting of misshapen perceptions, will add immeasurably to the quality of life. If one cannot achieve a modicum of success independently, medical help, with a heavy emphasis on psychotherapy, will be necessary.

ATTITUDINAL CHANGES AND PERSPECTIVE

Another method to reduce stress is to reinterpret it. Stress is a gift of life. It is an indication that you are a full participant of the grand drama of life. Its imperfections, challenges and perils should be viewed as opportunities. Every threatening event represents an extraordinary opportunity to change course, do better or consider options that would never have been envisaged otherwise. One may be compelled to find better solutions, to explore more productive avenues and break out of stifling routines. The benefit: the aggrandizing and energizing effect of success. Stress is not just a challenge, it is an open invitation to thrive. Welcome it! Thrive on it!

Keeping things in perspective is a major constituent of wisdom with the upshot of diffusing the noxious aspects of the stress reaction. Stand back, remove yourself from the microscopic aspect of a given dilemma and look at it from the perspective of the large picture. Are those daily irritants, put in proper perspective, really worth losing sleep over? It is so easy to get engrossed with minor inconveniences and lose sight of the grand scheme. Train yourself to disentangle your emotions from the grip of the moment to raise the unencumbered issue against the backdrop of your life's master plan.

RESPONSIBLE LIVING

The essence of responsible living is the artful decision-making that matches your major life choices with your capabilities and your natural inclinations. The better the match, the less opportunity there will be for conflict or unmet expectations and, therefore, stress. This idea cannot be over-emphasized: the major responsibility to yourself is to define your capabilities and work within their natural limits. This does not eliminate stress altogether but it sure diminishes its density.

STRESS LOAD REDUCTION

The most effective way to reduce stress levels, accessible to anyone, is to make wise and responsible choices. Not in the nitty-gritty details of everyday living, but in the major orientations of one's life. As already mentioned, the key is matching the endeavour with the competence.

■ Educational Choices

The more knowledge you assimilate, the better. A superior understanding of life, a higher socio-economic status, greater self-esteem are but a few of the advantages of a higher education and they are all conducive to avoiding life's worst stresses. Knowledge is power, knowledge is aptitude, knowledge is the dissipation of irrational fears, knowledge is happiness, knowledge is energy.

■   Vocational Choices

A career choice well-matched to your native intelligence, educational level, personality and personal interests will most assuredly reduce the incidence of stress-producing circumstances.

■   Marital Choice

The right choice of spouse is crucial. While there is not much argument about this simple fact, the difficult part is making that perfect choice. Choice implies discrimination. Discrimination implies a large enough sample to put it into effect. If you can screen one thousand candidates versus two or three, chances are you will find a superior match. One aspect, therefore, of the selection process, is the availability of a broad spectrum of options. How? Plunge into the hurly-burly of society and engage in as many social activities as your time and energy will permit. The more people you come in contact with, the better your selection.

How do you decide who is your best choice? Don't entrust that job to your "brain" (cognitive center). It is rather incompetent in this area. Entrust it to your heart (limbic areas of the central nervous system). The intensity of love is the evolutionary paradigm that has guided the animal species for three or so billion years. It knows exactly what to do. Trust your sense of love. There is a natural proportionality between intensity of love and appropriateness (biological) of the match. The final point on this issue is the importance of similarity. The more similar your mate is to you, the greater the chances of success and, conversely, the poorer the match, the greater the risk of conflict and stress. Similarity of race, culture, religion, phenotype (physical genetic expression), temperament, personality, socio-economic status, educational level, interests and so on, is of great benefit. Don't believe that opposites attract! In fact, they clash.

■   Avoidance of Aberrant Lifestyles

Can you imagine a more stressful existence than an 18-year-old single mother on welfare, addicted to crack cocaine, prostituting herself to make ends meet only to end up in jail for a criminal act? The obvious message is that you are begging for stress overload if you engage in: (1) illegal activities, (2) immoral activities, (3) unhealthy habits, (4) substance abuse, (5) a self-centered egotistical approach to life.

■ Micro-management of Stress Load Reduction

Everyone's daily activities are peppered with minor irritants that in the aggregate might be significant wasters of energy. These inevitable irritants are usually quite specific for a given individual and entirely subjective in their impact. The supplicant is the only one able to gauge them and devise ways of eliminating them. These daily stresses are like weeds in an otherwise beautiful lawn. The more successful you are in plucking them out, the more beautiful and healthy the lawn is. Each one of us should identify these weeds (daily stresses) and eradicate them. Slowly, but surely, with astute stress management, your comfort level will rise significantly. You will be dumbfounded to discover how very simple changes in one's life can have such a dramatic effect on stress reduction.

LIVE AUTHENTICALLY

Your behavior, your image and your pursuits must be in harmony with your inner reality. To believe one thing and act out another is a recipe for conflict and stress. To act out an artificial self a la Hollywood will eventually wear you down. Your must accept yourself, love yourself and have the courage to show the world yourself - warts and all. Spending an undue amount of time and energy to hide non-malleable imperfections is a waste. Not worth it. Counterproductive. It will only turn on you and bite you. Remove falsehoods, expose yourself undisguised, and you will find humility, serenity and a genuine love of yourself.

TECHNIQUES TO ENHANCE STRESS RESISTANCE

Stress must be managed effectively for survival, and even more so for thriving. Different types of stresses require different approaches. Add to this the huge subjective component of any challenge, and you will acknowledge that there is no universal formula to manage stress. One should adopt many synergistic methods to enhance the chances of success. The mission is very much similar to an army general's whose army is just about to face a formidable enemy and engage in a life and death battle. How would you prepare? You would attempt to assemble a group of strong, healthy and well-equipped soldiers fully trained for the mission, gain an accurate assessment of the enemy's strengths, weaknesses and vulnerable areas, summon additional help if the enemy is too powerful, possibly flee, if the enemy is undefeatable or the cost of battle is too high, and employ every known technique to reassure, motivate, energize and instill belief in the troops. The battle against stress is no different. The following are universally attainable coping methods:

(1) Increase your Resistance to Stress

Your state of physical and mental health will have an enormous influence on your vulnerability to stress. If you are emotionally drained, fatigued, or ill, your ability to cope with stress is diminished. Financial, societal and marital strength conversely will provide a cushion against the onslaught of stressful events. A financial loss of $10,000 would be inconsequential for the millionaire but devastating for the unemployed on the edge of bankruptcy. The best protection against adversity is to make yourself impervious through optimizing and toughening up every important facet of your life:

- make yourself healthy, strong and well-rested
- learn emotional control and balance
- invest in your general knowledge fund
- establish an extensive support system with family and friends
- acquire adequate financial resources to meet unexpected downturns

Strength is a most potent antidote to stress.

(2) Expand your Knowledge Base

Ignorance breeds fear. Misunderstandings, misjudgments, inaccurate facts, fear of the unknown, will convert inherently benign happenings into distressing experiences. Just contrast the reaction of a young child and a mature adult to a loud thundering roar during a storm. The child, because of lack of precise knowledge, will imagine the worst and experience extreme fear. The mature adult who understands the workings of nature and has experienced these events in the past (and therefore clued in as to their benignity), will hardly react at all. This same gap in magnitude of stress reaction is true for almost all life's challenges. Knowledge is the ultimate anti-stressor. Its possession opens the mind to all possible solutions.

(3) Conditioning

We all develop reflexes to various stimuli. Certain patterns of response, through repeated re-enactment, become imprinted and automatic. Mental reflexes are just as real as the familiar physical ones.

Can one establish positive mental reflexes such as optimism, positive thinking and ambition? Absolutely, but it doesn't come easy. To establish a mental reflex one must alter the connections between neurons (dendrites) in a very specific way. This process is called plasticity. It is slow and can only be activated through intense repetition. Eventually, through obstinate rehearsal, new attitudes and patterns of response will emerge.

A simple example will serve to illustrate the stress-reducing potential of positive thinking. Consider your spouse. If you keep obsessing on his or her bad points, they soon dominate your consciousness, and life with him or her becomes intolerable. If, on the other hand, you suppress the irritants and concentrate on the good points, then your spouse becomes a wonderful partner. Your perceptual reflexes minimize the negative and maximize the positive. The difference? Same people but better attitudes, less stress, less unhappiness and less fatigue.

(4) Desensitization

An anxiety-ridden activity can become quite tolerable and, occasionally, frankly enjoyable, by exploiting the biological phenomenon of desensitization. With repeated exposures associated with a benign outcome, one will become less and less physically reactive and, eventually, the experience becomes entirely tolerable. Through this desensitization, our neuro-hormonal stress responses diminish, our receptors down-regulate and, thus, we become accustomed to these specific stressful events.

Many of our stressors can be subdued in this way. One takes a pro-active stance, increases the frequency and intensity of the exposure to specific stressful events to eventually "get used to it", i.e. to become desensitized.

Public speaking is a good example. This is universally stressful. However, the more you do it, the easier it gets and the less stressful it becomes. You can desensitize yourself progressively to the point of complete comfort. If you are destined to perform stressful duties at regular intervals, like public speaking, a strategy of desensitization makes sense. This is applicable to a whole variety of activities ranging from sitting alone in a cafeteria, meeting new people, fear of elevators, to chairing staff meetings.

(5) Prioritization

Yes, you have ten things to do and only time for five. Don't double your work time - do only what you can. Prioritize and pace yourself. Over the long-term, any other *modus operandi* will exact a heavy price. Nothing is so critical that it cannot be postponed or left aside or assigned to someone else. We only think it is; it never is. If your boss wants you to do more than you can comfortably cope with, sit down with him and seek his opinion on priorities. Get him or her involved in that decision-making process. The boss will realize your conundrum and his tacit approval of the agreed-upon priorities will greatly alleviate your stress.

Delegation is a wonderful blow-off valve and should be exploited to the maximum. Why should you do everything and get exhausted in the process? Spread the work around. My wife discovered this principle very early in our marriage.

(6) Humour

Humour is a potent anti-stressor. Make a point of observing how often people engage in humour when faced with a very stressful duty. Their intuition or natural reflex is absolutely correct. Humour diminishes fear, anxiety and has a relaxing effect. The next time you attend a lecture or a conference, observe the speaker before he/she gives the talk. You will be amazed at how often he/she engages in light-hearted conversation or will start the lecture with a joke or humourous comment.

Humour has a way of alleviating fear, diminishing the apparent magnitude of the perceived threat and taking the edge off the physical manifestations of stress. There is nothing more calming than to inject humour in any particularly difficult human interaction. Not only does humour make your opponent less daunting, but it also makes you less threatening and, therefore, less likely to trigger aggressive-defensive reactions from your opponent. Double benefit!

(7) Automatisms

Hate housework? Can't stand humdrum chores? Can't afford to get it done by somebody else? Remove the emotional content: just do it systematically, unvaryingly, efficiently and predictably. Don't think about it. Do it automatically and think of something else. If you can organize your week in such a way that the bulk of your unpleasant or stressful chores are consolidated and done unemotionally and automatically, stress levels will abate. Disconnect your emotions and let automatism take over.

(8) Friendship

Isolation is an ally of stress. It will magnify the threat, distort it and deny the victim the benefits of friendly advice and reality checks. Support systems, especially family and close friends, are extremely important in the battle against stress in general. Talking, ventilating - even ranting - is positively helpful; you also profit from the corrective effect of somebody else's viewpoint. It is so reassuring to have a friend tell you the mountain is a mole hill and to chill out! An astute friend may find, within the maze of life's predicaments, the genial solution liable to turn your life around. Friendship is an extraordinary shield against stress in general.

(9)   Spirituality

The spiritual dimension is a valuable perspective through which problems may be filtered. Your religious conviction is a first-line stand against stress. Picture the benefits:

- God showers you with unconditional love
- God confers upon you significance and self-esteem
- God provides you with an ultimate destination
- God's moral code reduces the stress of choices which, in turn, promotes peace of mind
- God's teachings point to a healthful lifestyle conducive to creating a stress-free path in life
- God provides every ingredient for success
- guaranteed survival making death a mere transition
- there is a pot of gold at the end of the line (eternal happiness in heaven) which makes life's problems mere peccadillos considering the ultimate prize

There is no question that an unmitigated belief in religious tenets has an extraordinary impact on stress levels. If you hold that genuine belief and act on it, you are in a very fortunate position.

(10)   Flight

If you find yourself in an irretrievably nightmarish marriage, if you live in a dangerous environment, if your job is making you totally miserable, if your responsibilities overwhelm you and, if you realistically can't do much about it, then retreat. Fleeing is a survival scheme, not cowardice. You have to know when you are beat! David and Goliath is a cute little story, but in reality, David would get crushed in one second flat. Recognize the indomitable or the irreconcilable and flee it.

(11)   Physical Relaxation

Relaxation produces physiologic effects opposite to those of stress. It slows the heart rate, respiratory rate, lowers the blood pressure, increases peripheral blood flow and restores neuromuscular stability. Stress reactions are muted by relaxation techniques.

Most techniques include progressive muscular relaxation, from head to toe, in sequential order. Relaxation is further encouraged by soothing tape-recorded messages or music.

Mental imagery of secure, cuddly and utterly pleasant environments fosters a state of muscular and physiologic untightening. Massages, sighing, stretching, hot baths and exercise, will also promote unwinding.

Relaxation not only opposes the physiologic responses to stress, it also breaks a vicious circle. The perception of a pounding heart, rapid breathing, sweating and shaking extremities, reinforces the anxiety of a stressful event. Relaxation mutes the physical manifestations of stress and breaks this vicious circle.

(12) The Power of Inner Talk

We all talk to ourselves. Our brain is a veritable chatter-box. It is a wonderful way to sort out our problems, and find solutions. Inner talk is an extremely powerful weapon in the arsenal of stress management. It helps to reconcile ourselves with reality, to inject perspective on the issue, to dissect problems into its basic elements, to plan and implement a strategic solution, to calm yourself, to reassure yourself, and provides an inner forum for the assessment of your progress. Inner talk can be best incorporated with your daily walks (walk the dog!). In no time will you reap the purgative benefits on the soul. If you systematically repress negative attitudinal reflexes, adjust perception for more objectivity and draw from your well-honed knowledge-based wisdom the genius of problem-solving, you have stress licked.

(13) Know When to Seek Help

You are not Superman. If you are unfortunate enough to be in an unfavorable environment, and genetically vulnerable, stress may be overwhelming. There might come a time when you are unable to cope with it. The recognition is usually quite straightforward: constant anxiety, depression, burn-out, loss of physical well-being, among others. These symptoms should compel you to get help. An ever-present danger is the tendency to develop compensatory bad habits as a coping mechanism. Alcoholism, drug addition, aberrant lifestyles are obvious examples.

What is less obvious is the risk of developing distorted views of reality in a futile attempt of converting painful circumstances into more tolerable conditions. These distorted views of reality are a result of the overuse of perfectly normal defense mechanisms. Overuse of these defense mechanisms is a sign of not coping. While most defense mechanisms are useful, short-term, and in small dosages, complications arise when they become established patterns of behavior. This type of mental conditioning is pernicious in the long run. The sooner you recognize this insidious transformation the better; it is an indication to seek help. Defense mechanisms to recognize:

-   Denial: negating external reality because it is too painful
-   Distortion: reshaping external reality to suit inner needs, i.e. delusion
-   Primitive idealization: objects are unrealistically endowed with great power
-   Projection: unacceptable inner impulses are attributed to someone else and reacted to as though they were outside the self
-   Splitting: repetitive oscillation between contradictory self-concepts, i.e. one day you are all good and, another, all bad
-   Acting out: giving in to a fanciful impulse
-   Hypochondriasis: self-reproach is translated into complaints of pain, illness and weakness to avoid responsibility or guilt
-   Identification: transforming oneself into a loved one, admired one, or an aggressor, either for self-punitive purposes or to mitigate separation anxiety
-   Introjection: internalization of the qualities of an object; it obliterates the difference between the subject and the object
-   Passive-aggressive behavior: aggression is expressed indirectly through passivity, masochism and turning against the self

- Regression: return to an earlier phase of personality development to avoid the tension and conflict at the present level of development
- Schizoid fantasy: autistic retreat into fantasy to resolve conflicts and to avoid intimacy
- Somatization: psychic conflicts are converted into bodily symptoms
- Controlling: excessive attempt to control to reduce anxiety
- Displacement: symbolic representation
- Dissociation: drastic transmutation of a personal identity to avoid emotional distress
- Externalization: tendency to perceive in the external world, elements of one's own personality
- Inhibition: repression of ego functions
- Intellectualization: excessive use of intellectual processes to avoid affective expressions or experiences
- Isolation: separating an idea from its effect
- Rationalization: rational explanations to justify unacceptable attitudes, beliefs or behavior
- Reaction formation: an unacceptable impulse is transformed into its opposite
- Repression: curbing ideas and feelings before attaining consciousness
- Sexualization: projection of sexual significance to objective events
- Ascetism: elimination of life's pleasures
- Suppression: postponement of attention to a conflict

(14) Learn to Say "No"

It is intimidating to say no. We fear retaliation arising from hurt feelings. Our sense of obligation is sometimes inappropriate. We think of innumerable reasons for acquiescing to unpleasant chores. When excessive stress is an issue, and when you are truly overloaded with work, just say no. You have to learn to simply say no. Surprisingly, you will realize that more often than not, you gain in respect. Fear of retaliation is not a realistic feeling when the reason for the refusal is legitimate. It is a baseless anxiety.

CHAPTER 9
WHEN THE PROBLEM IS YOUR LIFESTYLE

Lifestyle is an all-encompassing term that includes the quantity, diversity, intensity, character and quality of every component of our daily routine. We adopt lifestyles to satisfy personal, interpersonal and societal needs. Unfortunately, our ability to interpret our needs is frequently limited and countless imperfections and frank aberrations may quietly set in. To compound the quandary, we are not infrequently forgetful of our limitations and weaknesses. Unhealthy lifestyles will result in abnormal fatigue. Either they starve an overworked machinery or simply overwhelm its operating limits.

One major component of a lifestyle may be at fault and be the sole reason for asthenia (i.e. running daily marathons) or, as is much more frequent, there are innumerable small contributors. An objective analysis of our lifestyle could ferret out hidden vices that interfere with optimal function. Once detected, it is generally easy to correct them

ABSENCE OF EQUILIBRIUM

Excess of anything and the deficiency of essential ingredients in a frenetic lifestyle are the most common sins. In North America, the pursuit of money or fame has spawned workaholism, a by-product of capitalism and a prime symptom of unchecked ambitions and compensatory behaviour. Too much work and too little of everything else is a recipe for burnout and fatigue.

The various excesses that will lead to fatigue either singly or in combination are:
. excess work
. excess exercise
, excess sports
. excess sex
. excess romance
. excess food
. excess alcohol
. excessive smoking

A biological equilibrium is essential. The specific point of that equilibrium in any given individual should be determined either by trial and error or using broad averages of normal habitual human behavior. If common sense and experimentation don't work, then professional counseling is in order.

Leisure time is a *sine qua non*. The mission, however, is delicate. The wrong choice of leisure activity can be counter-productive. For example, competitive sports or aggressive chess-playing are not restful. Leisure time must almost be boring to qualify. Easy-going, non stimulating and soothing activities such as easy-listening music, walking the dog, light T.V. programs, are necessary for a proper regenerative respite.

LIFESTYLE BLIGHTS

Chronic dislikes act like a cancer and shunt away valuable energy. Major aversions in the living environment should be extirpated. These can range from a terrible job, obnoxious acquaintances, depressing apartment, dangerous neighborhood, disastrous marriage etc. Whatever the cancer may be, it should be resected sooner rather than later. Otherwise it will drain the lifeblood out of you.

ENERGY WASTERS

Every once in a while, one should analyze a typical day's activities from the first second of wakefulness to the last minute before sleep and weed out the activities that are unimportant, purposeless or too costly in terms of energy consumption for what they produce. Long commutes, disorganization, hustle and bustle, rush-hour driving, perfectionistic rituals, inefficient methods (washing dishes instead of using a dishwasher), fidgetiness, refusing to delegate, inability to say no (taxiing the kids around twenty times/day), tackling jobs for which you are totally incompetent (e.g. plumbing), pointless arguments are but a few examples of what your might find. If you systematically weed out energy wasters, you will be left with more energy to enjoy.

UNHEALTHY HABITS

Any habit that degrades your general health, directly or indirectly, reduces the optimal functioning of your body and thereby lowers the threshold for fatigue. This general principle holds true for just about anything that detracts from perfect health. Cigarette smoking, immoderate amounts of alcohol, illegal drugs, excessive food intake, wrong foods, poor hygiene, sedentary lifestyle, exposure to pollutants are significant vitiators of good health and will exacerbate chronic fatigue. The more one can upgrade general health, the more one will be resistant to fatigue.

UNLAWFUL BEHAVIOR

The breach of laws, be they political, natural, social or religious, as an inherent feature of one's lifestyle, is a recipe for disaster. Invariably, the law-breaker assumes that he will get away with it. Chances are he won't. There is always a price to pay.

Let's look at the downside of systematic law-breaking.

. the "tension" attending the possibility of getting caught or being exposed
. the complicated web of deceit to keep unlawful activities well hidden
. the inevitable circumstances where the illegal or immoral actions are threatening exposure with the associated extreme anxiety
. constant background worry
. constant background guilt
. degradation of general health
. loss of self-esteem
. disappointment with the ill-gotten gains
. compensatory aberrant behavior
. greater difficulty relaxing
. risk of poorer sleep

One way or the other, you pay the price. One of them is chronic fatigue. This principle applies to the whole spectrum of illicit behaviors: from white collar fraud, to marital infidelity, to malfeasance against our fellow man. Inevitable in these ventures is the debilitating side-effect of energy wastage for illusory gains. In the grand scheme of things, unethical, unlawful or unnatural behavior does not pay off. Sin is fatiguing.

ALTERNATIVE LIFESTYLES

If you analyze the history of mankind and decipher the underlying reason for social conflict, you will probably come to the conclusion that the essential ingredient is dissimilarity. Dissimilarity in race, culture, language, dress, color, religious beliefs, sexual mores, lifestyles, economics, politics, you name it. The mere presence of non-conformity invites conflict and strife. For biological reasons, human beings dislike dissimilarity and perceive it as a threat. Whatever the explanation is, the practical point is that the more you differ, the more you contrast and the more you rub against the cultural grain of a society, the more you invite intolerance. The more social resistance you encounter, the more stress you endure and the more energy you consume. Everything else being equal, you will suffer more intense fatigue.

To adopt an alternative lifestyle, there should be a solid purpose. Oddballs, eccentric personalities, over-decorated walking billboards, pierced everything, purple hair, provocative dressing and so on might be very entertaining but rather counter-productive. Non-conformity carries a heavy price, so evaluate the benefits carefully before indulging. If you are on the edge of disabling chronic fatigue, you probably won't tolerate the deprecating attention.

CHAPTER 10
WHEN THE BASICS OF
HEALTHFUL LIVING ARE AT FAULT

These basics are sleep, exercise and proper nutrition. All three play significant roles not only in general health but in the decisive campaign against incapacitating fatigue. The most important one is, not surprisingly, sleep. The absence of sufficient regenerative rest is the pivot around which revolves all other issues. This critical area of human physiology will be discussed at length because it alone will make or break any comprehensive program to overcome fatigue.

SLEEP

We spend one-third of our life sleeping. The impulse to sleep is triggered by fatigue, and when we enact this mysterious physiological imperative, we awake regenerated and recharged to take on the day. Sleep is not unique to human beings, it impels every living creature on the planet. It's universality stamps it as a fundamental need of organic existence. The recuperative function of sleep is indisputable. What remains largely unknown is how it does it. Energy balance, cellular integrity, consolidation of central nervous system acquisitions (memory), repair processes are all enabled by this complex state that is sleep. Sleep is not static! It goes through numerous neurophysiological transformations, each critical to the restorative process.

Rest or sleep does not mean stoppage of activity. In fact, there is no organ system that suspends its activities. There is a progressive diminution in the rate of work of most cellular functions, the most relevant being the central nervous system neurons.

The sleeping brain goes through five phases, each recognizable with EEG tracings (measures the brain's electrical activity). There is slow-wave sleep (4 stages) and REM sleep (characterized by rapid eye movements). Slow-wave sleep evolves through four stages of deepening unconsciousness and associated physiological changes over a period of 30 to 45 minutes. About every 90 minutes, slow-wave sleep converts to a different form of sleep called REM sleep. This stage is recognized by the rapid phasic contractions of the eye muscles, causing the eyes to cyclically shift from side to side. Dreams occur during this phase of sleep.

What does the brain do when asleep?
- consciousness is progressively depressed
- intellectual functions are suspended
- emotional centers are uncoupled
- autonomic nervous system centers diminish their activity
- motor and sensory functions are largely suspended
- consolidation of learning
- most nerve cells remain quite active electrically even though their efferent effects are absent - this uncoupling suggests that these cells are actively "restoring" themselves.
- dreaming; the purpose of which is still unknown

Other systems in the body also adjust their activities:

- some hormones increase (growth hormone) and some diminish (catecholamines)
- all muscles relax
- sensory organs shut-down (vision, taste etc)
- heart rate and blood pressure decrease
- breathing slows
- body temperature decreases
- gastro-intestinal motility increases

The whole gamut of sleep-related functions can fill text books; one needs to only remember that sleep is basically restorative. Absence of sufficient sleep or absence of any portion of its cascade leads to serious dysfunction and, ultimately, breakdown and death. It is the center piece in the arsenal to fight fatigue.

The consequences of insufficient sleep or poor quality sleep are grave:

- fatigue
- constant urge to doze off
- diminishes the performance of many bodily systems: dulls the brain, accident proneness, depletes the immune defense system, promotes growth of fat instead of muscle, accelerates ageing, impairs memory
- increases stress hormones
- spoils human relationships
- exacerbates depression

With severe sleep deprivation:

- hallucinations
- irritability
- difficulty in concentrating
- episodes of disorientation
- prolonged insomnia is fatal (in animals)

With dysfunction of certain sleep stages:

- sleep-walking
- bed-wetting
- night terror
- nightmares

. sleep-related seizures
. teeth grinding

Sleep requirements are not negotiable. Like it or not, you are genetically programmed to comply with, on average, approximately eight hours of good quality sleep. Variances of roughly two hours on either side are not unusual. With age, sleep requirements diminish. Habitual sleep duration of fewer than four hours or greater than nine, is associated with increased mortality rates as compared to sleep durations of seven to eight hours per night.

SLEEP DISTURBANCES

One-third of adults in the United States experience occasional or persistent sleep disturbances. Sleep deprivation that is not naturally explicable, or that persists for three weeks or more, should trigger medical consultation. Table 10.1 will give you an inkling of the conditions your doctor will consider during his clinical evaluation. If your doctor discovers poor sleep habits, an aberrant lifestyle, psychological or psychiatric problems or a specific medical condition, he will take the necessary steps to remedy the situation. For certain conditions (i.e. sleep apnea) he may refer you to a sleep specialist.

A condition which is highly under-diagnosed, especially in its mild form, is the sleep-apnea syndrome. This condition is very important because it is prevalent, difficult to diagnose, has profound repercussions on daytime alertness and quality of life, and is treatable.

Sleep-apnea syndrome is a condition where breathing becomes obstructed (air flow into the lung literally stops) during deep sleep and, as it persists, triggers arousal or partial awakening so as to resume normal unobstructed breathing. If one observes an episode of obstructed breathing, it is obvious that the individual makes an effort to breathe but nothing gets through; a block occurs in the upper airway (throat). The recurrent arousal triggered by the near-asphyxiating effects of respiratory obstruction cumulatively depletes deep sleep. Thus, a state of sleep deprivation develops.

The mechanism of sleep-apnea is known. During the deepest stages of sleep, the muscles in the upper airway relax and collapse the airway. Persons with narrow airways are particularly prone to this obstruction because there is less room to spare. Several factors promote upper airway collapse during sleep. Obesity, recessed chin, enlarged tongue (hypothyroidism), large uvula and soft palate (small tongue of tissue hanging at the back of the throat), large tonsils/adenoids, nasal obstruction, excess alcohol intake, cigarette smoking, and a family history of hypertension, are the main ones.

TABLE 10.1
CONDITIONS THAT INTERFERE WITH SLEEP

NARCOLEPSY	NOCTURNAL TERROR, CRAMPS, ENURESIS
PSYCHOLOGICAL	NIGHTMARES
SLEEP-APNEA SYNDROME	NEURO-DEGENERATIVE DISORDERS
RESTLESS LEG SYNDROME	PARKINSON'S DISEASE
POOR SLEEPING HABITS	SLEEP-RELATED EPILEPSY
DISTURBING ENVIRONMENT	SLEEP-RELATED HEADACHES
HIGH ALTITUDE INSOMNIA	NOCTURNAL ANGINA OR DYSPPNEA
FOOD ALLERGY INSOMNIA	CHRONIC OBSTRUCTIVE LUNG DISEASE
INSOMNIA RELATED TO DRUGS OR ALCOHOL	SLEEP-RELATED ASTHMA
JET LAG, SHIFT WORK, LATE OR EARLY PHASES SLEEP	GASTRO-DUODENAL ULCER DISEASE
GASTRO-INTESTINAL REFLUX	FIBROSITIS SYNDROME
ATYPICAL SLEEP CYCLES	ANY CHRONIC PAIN

There are clues to this condition, the most important ones being the observations made by the sleep-mate:

- chronic snoring (partial obstruction)
- witnessed apnea (non-breathing) and/or choking
- frequent awakenings
- unrefreshing sleep
- excessive daytime sleepiness
- poor memory
- irritability
- nocturia (nocturnal urination)
- diminished sex drive
- morning headaches

Many of these symptoms are non-specific, so the diagnosis rests on a high index of suspicion.

The aim of treatment is the relief of apnea. Measures such as weight loss, smoking cessation and avoidance of nocturnal sedation (especially alcohol) may be beneficial. Treatment possibilities include: tongue repositories, mandibular positioners, CPAP (a tight-fitting mask to administer continuous positive airway pressure) and upper airway surgery, such as uvulopalatopharyngoplasty.

STRATEGIES TO OPTIMIZE SLEEP

Investing in the prerequisites of a sound and regenerative sleep is a highly profitable undertaking. A well-rested, refreshed individual will almost invariably be a happier person. There is, however, no magic formula to guarantee optimal sleep. Like everything else in life, there is a host of small factors which individually may seem insignificant, but, cumulatively, have a major impact on sleep quality. The following recommendations are conducive to proper sleeping and provide a basic strategic framework.

(1) Rule Out a Medical Problem

As already discussed, if there is any doubt about the presence of an underlying medical problem. Consult your physician. This is particularly pertinent if the quality of your sleep has been suffering for a long period of time (greater than 3-4 weeks) or if insomnia recurs frequently (3-4 times per year).

(2)   Trust your Instincts

Sleep requirements are genetically-programmed. Your biological clock is not negotiable. Your intuition is the most competent guide in determining the length and timing of sleep. Listen to it - it knows best. If you are drowsy and nodding off, it is nature's indication of tiredness and it's time to sleep. Very simple and straightforward. If you feel good and refreshed with eight hours of sleep and not quite so with only seven hours, you need an additional hour of sleep. If you feel great and operate optimally after six hours of sleep then good for you and enjoy it. Personal monitoring over a sufficient period of time will indicate your body's needs. No other method will give a more accurate reading of your natural sleep requirements.

Don't even dream of cheating on your sleep quota. Any accumulated deficit will inevitably have to be paid. Your central nervous system keeps a running balance on your "sleep account" and will never let you off the hook. Chronic fatigue, general underperformance and increased risk of illness is the price to pay for running a chronic sleep deficit.

Had a particularly good night's sleep and felt absolutely fantastic the next day? Keep a diary of all the possible factors that played a role in creating the setting for that wonderful sleep. Over time, common denominators may surface and could be exploited profitably for the rest of your life. Even details that, at first blush, might seem insignificant may turn out to be effective sleep promoters.

The converse is also useful. Keep track of all the factors that went into giving you that dreadful night's sleep. You will definitely want to avoid these.

(3)   Turn Off the Alertness Switch

Alertness is the antithesis of sleepiness. They represent extreme poles of the biological rhythm called circadian rhythm. Daytime alertness and nighttime sleepiness go through precise 24-hour cycles along with many other circadian rhythms. Alertness is the optimal activated state of the brain required for peak performance.

All the switches that stimulate and sustain alertness are precisely the ones that need to be turned off for sleep induction. As the day wears on, one should progressively diminish the stimuli that stoke the fires of alertness.

■ Stimulating Thoughts

A sense of danger, a peaked interest or an alluring opportunity, fear, anxiety, an anger-provoking thought - all will stimulate the sympathetic nervous system which places the brain in full alert. For at least an hour before bedtime, these thoughts and/or emotions should be resolutely suppressed. Mentally eradicate them. Any tendency for those rousing thoughts to re-emerge in your consciousness should be met with an iron-fisted will to suppress them.

■ Muscular Activity

The last hour of the day should be one of relaxation. Exercise, even mild exercise, has a stimulating effect and therefore should be avoided late in the day. Strenuous exercise should not be envisaged for at least three hours before bedtime.

■ Time of Day on the Circadian Clock

Keep a regular time for sleeping in tune with your biological clock. Constant out of phase sleeping times, either too early or too late, will wreak havoc on sleep induction. Jet lag, shift work, late night carousing, are physiologically stressful and trigger costly regulatory adjustments that take time and energy. There is a wealth of information available on the damaging effects of poorly-planned and poorly-managed shift work schedules in industry. Cyclical shift workers should consult an expert in the field to manage this very specific predicament.

■ Food and Chemicals

Snacking, caffeine, nicotine and a variety of drugs may intensify alertness and thus interfere with sleep induction. A heavy, late-evening snack, consumption of coffee, tea, carbonated drinks, chocolate (caffeine), cigarette smoking and the ingestion of amphet-amine-like drugs, are all conducive to poor or restless sleep. Those who are particularly sensitive to caffeine should avoid its consumption for a good eight hours before sleep. Chocolate is not often recognized as a culprit. Not only does it contain caffeine, but also bromides (related to amphetamines), which are stimulants.

■ Light

Brightness (bright lights) suppresses sleep and increases alertness. Darkness promotes the reverse.

■ Sound

Smooth, continuous sound, such as rolling surf or a mountain stream, is relaxing and a good sleep promoter. Irregular or choppy sounds will agitate you. A creaky door that intermittently shifts, a dripping faucet, a chiming grandfather clock and wind sounds will wreak havoc on your night's sleep. Avoid them just as you would (avoid) sand in your food.

■ Temperature

A cool room to reduce body temperature is conducive to sleep but the sensation of cold air against the skin increases alertness. You should find the right compromise. The converse applies to warmth.

Sleep is encouraged by a <u>fall</u> in body temperature. Consequently, activities that raise body temperature should be scheduled so as to precede bedtime by a long enough latent period to synchronize the fall in body temperature with sleep induction. Thus, a hot water bath should be taken approximately 90 minutes before bedtime and a session of exercise 3-4 hours before attempting to sleep.

(4) Idealize the Sleep Environment

The bedroom environment should be a shrine to the God of Sleep, Morpheus. All aspects of physical comfort should be contrived and maintained that way. The last items you want to skimp on in your budget is pillows and mattresses. Get the very best within your means.

The room should be familiar, secure, perfectly dark, perfectly quiet, and cool. The pillows should be exactly as you want them and the mattress should be near perfection for comfort.

Check every decorative aspect of your room and turn it into a haven of tranquility and comfort. You are the ultimate judge of what enhances your sleep performance and what detracts from it. If your partner snores like an old tractor and is making you deaf and dumb, find a solution. Either the partner finds a cure for the disorder or sleeps in a separate bedroom.

(5) Exercise

An exercise program is a great adjunct to good sleep strategies. As an integral part of a total health program, exercise will make you healthier, happier, more relaxed, less stressed and, in a non-specific way, be conducive to quality sleep. As previously mentioned, a fall in body temperature encourages sleep induction. Early morning exercise as it is too remote from bedtime for that purpose. Late evening exercise is too stimulative and, therefore, may become counterproductive. The best time for exercise is 3-4 hours before bedtime, thus synchronizing the projected fall in body temperature with the onset of sleep. Intense exercise requires a longer latent period, perhaps up to 8 hours or more.

(6) Mental Conditioning

Conditioning is a double-edged sword. Positive conditioning borne out of a meticulously planned regular routine reinforces all the reflexes that go into promoting good sleep. There is, however, the risk of negative conditioning. The person who, after an experience with sleepless nights, becomes obsessed with the issue, can find himself embarking on a vicious circle: the anxiety provoked by the fear of losing sleep in itself promotes sleeplessness. This vicious circle can be broken by reassuring self-talk and eliminating all visual cues as to what time it is. The key is to realize that a sleepless night or two always feels worse than what it actually is (we sleep a lot more than we realize), is perfectly harmless, a simple inconvenience that will eventually be made up and is a perfectly natural occurrence in all human beings.

Remove all clocks or any cues that will give you feedback information regarding the time of night. This is extremely helpful as these cues tend to intensify the state of anxiety.

(7) Sleeping Pills

Avoid sleeping pills scupulously. They are truly a trap of short-term gain for long-term pain. They should be reserved for exceptional circumstances and usually after consultation with a physician.

Sleeping pills are one of the most abused medications in America. Unfortunately, they are an alluring quick-fix to a common problem at a very high cost in terms of physical well-being. Sleeping pills are not conducive to a normal sleep pattern (you never feel quite "right" the next day) and cause next-day lassitude. They are extremely habit-forming and, finally, suffer the drawback of pharmacologic tolerance where an equal effect requires ever-increasing dosages. One can become seriously addicted to this class of medication and the weaning process is very slow and painful. Rebound insomnia, which is the natural result of withdrawal from these drugs, is a powerful hook that compels the victim to return to its usage. The best approach is, like any other addiction, to not start in the first place. There are plenty of natural ways to tide you over a spell of insomnia. The popping of a sleeping pill should not be the first reaction.

Sleeping medications play a very important role in the medical arena with numerous established indications, but this is a far cry from the common usage as a convenient way to negotiate the lumps and bumps of life.

Alcohol should never be used as an hypnotic. Sure, you can drink yourself into an instantaneous coma but you will rise from the dead as soon as your blood alcohol levels wane. You will then wake up as "hyper" as ever, hung over, and destined for a totally miserable day. Not worth it!!

EXERCISE

An interesting paradox reveals itself in this area of human biology. Why would an activity which rapidly leads to a state of fatigue be helpful in combating a state of chronic fatigue? The answer to this question is extremely complex, primarily because there is so much science cannot explain (which is the underlying reason for most complex answers). There are many reasons why a sound exercise program is beneficial from a comprehensive health point-of-view and from an energy point-of-view. The most important one is anthropological.

Man is an evolutionary product of the animal species. He achieved this position after billions of years of adaptive biological transformations to meet environmental challenges. Life forms that have not successfully met these challenges have disappeared (99% of all life forms that ever emerged on earth). Man is a biological triumph.

Our immediate predecessors (apes) evolved biological systems that were equipped to meet average environmental demands. Exertional requirements to sustain life (i.e. hunting, foraging, fleeing predators, building shelter, body maintenance, competing for mates, migrating etc) moulded biological systems to cope with those demands. Every cell of the body ultimately evolved, capacitated to generate X amount of energy, consume Y amount of fuels and restore energetic balance with Z amount of rest. These energetic ranges are narrow, specific (i.e. muscle contraction) and relatively inflexible. Under-use an organ, cell or body system and it atrophies (reduces its mass and work capacity or strength). Overuse it and you trigger hypertrophy (increased mass, work capacity or strength). Overuse it or under-use it on a protracted basis and the tissue disintegrates (through complex biochemical abnormalities). Adaptive biology is unforgiving. Operate within these limits or else your body degrades. Figure 10.2 illustrates this principle.

If you under-exert yourself on average, you will suffer atrophy of the energy-producing machinery. This reduced capacity will lower the threshold for fatigue and greatly limit the scope of physical activities. If you over-exert on a protracted basis, you deplete energy stores and you damage the energy-producing machinery (inherent to the process of hypertrophy) and in this way also lower the threshold for fatigue. The proper range is right smack in between. The proper amount of total physical exertion must be in equilibrium with our inherited biological machinery and with our longstanding (1000s of years) environmental demands. Adaptation or evolution, however, is inherently slow (measured in thousands of years) and unpredictable.

Man's environment, particularly his technological environment, literally metamorphosed itself overnight. In a few hundred years, the efficiency of everyday living has exploded upwards in a staggering fashion. Modern modes of transportation, communications, food production, work appliances, enhanced security and so on have dramatically reduced the average exertional demands for survival. What may have been an exhausting task a few thousand years ago (putting food on the table) is virtually effortless today. The consequence of these extraordinary gains in efficiency is the emergence of a constant state of under-exertion relative to our biological machinery's specifications. A mismatch has occurred. The extraordinary gains in modern efficiency evidently outdistanced the biological evolutionary adjustments of the body. This disparity is most gaping in our locomotor apparatus (muscles, bones, joints, ligaments) and our cardiopulmonary system.

This unabating under-exertion leads to system atrophy, inefficiency and weakness.

The hypothesis then asserts itself. If one were to supplement this relatively sedentary lifestyle with just about the right amount of exercise to approximate the biological specifications (needs) of our body, then one would achieve optimal health, optimal strength, optimal efficiency and optimal efficacy. In this idealized state, the threshold for fatigue would be raised proportionately.

Dr. Claude R. Maranda

TABLE 10.2
EXERCISE AND FATIGUE

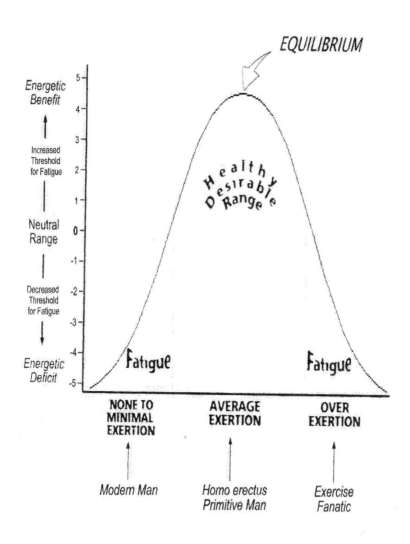

This hypothesis not only attempts to explain the desirability of exercise but also gives us a clue as to how much exercise is right for optimal health. Let's assume that primitive man (10,000 years ago), through evolution, was in energetic equilibrium with his environment. His sustained levels of physical exertion dictated by the imperatives of survival were within his biological operating limits. By estimating the amount of excess calories (convenient measure of work performed and energy consumed) expended over and above what a modern man would burn with his more efficient lifestyle, one would have a rough guide as to the magnitude of exercise supplementation necessary to restore the balance.

Primitive Man Versus Modern Man
Estimate of Daily Excess Caloric Expenditure
by Primitive Man

Activity	Total kcal/day
Personal hygiene	5
Walking	150
Running	40
Domestic chores	45
Miscellaneous work	40
Leisure, playing	20
	———
	300 kcal/day

Primitive man had to expend approximately 300 kcal/day more than modern man to accomplish his life-sustaining tasks. He had no car, no bicycle, no gun, nor a whole industry to prepare food for him. He did have to build a shelter and maintain his habitat. He did not have a TV to entertain himself, nor any books to read. Living was very much more physical and exceedingly less efficient.

From a purely empirical point-of-view, we can roughly estimate the amount by which we need to supplement our daily physical energy expenditure: approximately 300 kcal/day.

Table 10.3 gives examples of the "caloric currency" required to pay off this exercise debt.

Another element to factor in when assessing your exercise needs is the total daily caloric expenditure you customarily exact during regular work. If you are relatively sedentary, your needs are greater; but if you are very active (a construction worker, a mover, a postman), then exercise might be unnecessary and, in fact, counter-productive. Age must also be factored into the equation with the following adjustments:

Age	Kcal/day
10-30 years	350
31-50 years	300
51-70 years	250
71-90 years	200

A typical exercise prescription for a sedentary 40-year-old male could be: an average of 5 exercise sessions per week; an average of 400 kcal per session, comprised primarily of aerobic exercises.

One should attempt to exercise at least 3 days per week and include a minimum 2 days of rest per week. While the effect of exercise is cumulative in a given day, one should attempt to assign at least 20 minutes for continuous aerobic exercise. This is the threshold for a training effect.

The above exercise prescription is aggressive. Remember that it is designed for a completely sedentary individual. For any physical exertion, inherent to your work or lifestyle, you should deduct an equivalent amount in your exercise program

TABLE 10.3
CONSUMPTION OF 300 KCAL/DAY FOR A 70 KG MALE

Activity	Minutes per day
Badminton	42
Basketball	30
Canoeing	95

Carpentry	82
Carpet sweeping	88
Circuit-training	20
Cleaning	70
Cycling	40
Dancing	80
Digging trenches	26
Food shopping	70
Gardening	70
Golf	48
Ironing	65
Judo	20
Marching, rapid	28
Mopping floor	71
Piano playing	102
Painting	85
Running, slow	30
Running, fast	18
Scrubbing floors	38
Skiing	37
Snowshoeing	24
Swimming, crawl	30
Tennis	35
Volleyball	84
Walking, normal	50
Wallpapering	85
Window cleaning	70

Chronic fatigue sufferers are unlikely to tolerate an average exercise prescription, at least when the problem is at its worst. For any form of significant fatigue, one should double the conditioning period - 20 weeks instead of 10 - and halve the exercise duration and intensity. This only represents a rough guide. Every individual must determine his own tolerance level through trial and error.

PRECAUTIONS

While exercise confers immense benefits, it also has the capacity for harm. Table 10.4 lists the benefits and risks of concentrated exercise. As we can conclude from Table 10.4, exercise is a double-edged sword. If one is not careful, much harm may ensue. A reckless approach to exercise can convert a health enhancer into a liability. Several precautions are important. Observance of these will ensure a safe and productive endeavor.

(1) Medical Evaluation

If you are a male over 40 years of age, or a female over 50 years of age, if there is any suspicion of a health problem (in particular, cardiovascular), if there is the presence of one or more coronary risk factors (smoking, family history of "early" vascular disease, hypertension, diabetes, obesity, high cholesterol), you should consult your doctor for a medical evaluation. This may or may not include a stress test or an echocardiogram depending on the specific conclusions regarding your health risk. Not only is your risk evaluated, but your physician may also have suggestions for the types of exercises most suitable for you and the ones to avoid (i.e. jogging for an arthritic patient, weight-lifting for someone with hypertension). For an individual with coronary heart disease, a stress test is useful to determine up to what heart rate (an estimate of cardiac work) it is safe to exercise. Strict adherence to this limit reduces the chances of an untoward cardiac event.

Medical follow-up is advisable with specific medical problems where, as a result of a successful exercise program, adjustments in drug therapy are anticipated. Anti-hypertensives may be reduced, insulin requirements might decrease and, occasionally, antidepressants and anxiolytics might become unnecessary. Several health problems are ameliorated by judicious exercise and your physician will adjust therapy accordingly.

Pre-existent musculoskeletal problems should be assessed by a physician interested in this field to institute preventive measures with special equipment, customized sports shoes and so on.

TABLE 10.4
RISKS AND BENEFITS OF EXERCISE
BENEFITS   **RISKS**

Increased:

strength of muscles, tendons
and ligaments
stability of joints
balance and mobility
coordination
recreational pleasures
bone mass
sleep quality
cognitive functions
ventilatory capacity
oxygenation
fibrinolysis
heat tolerance
sexual function
self confidence
self-esteem
stress resistance
quality of life
physical beauty
energy
socialization
independence

Decreased:

risk of injury, falls, accidents
lipids (cholesterol, triglycerides)
blood pressure
heart attacks
other vascular diseases
constipation
glucose intolerance (diabetes)
stress hormones
colon and breast cancer
depression, anxiety
obesity
ageing

musculo-skeletal injury
arthritis
overuse syndromes
stress fracture
heart attack
arrhythmias
sudden death
aortic rupture
intracerebral bleeding
insomnia
sleepiness, fatigue
air pollution
diarrhea
low blood sugar
dehydration
diminished libido
amenorrhea
infertility
heartburn
hernias
barotrauma
nervousness
aggressivity
marital alienation
addiction
environmental risk (sunburn,
        frostbite)
expenses

116

(2) Exercise Wisdom

Whatever sport or exercise you adopt, make a point of learning everything about it. There are countless books in libraries or bookstores devoted to this subject. For most of us, professional guidance is not available or practical (or affordable) but if it is, by all means partake of it. Not only will your sporting activity be safer but more enjoyable.

Choose the right equipment. This is the last place to scrimp. For jogging you must wear the right shoes. For cycling you need the right bicycle. If you wish to roller-blade you should wear the right protective equipment. If you enjoy racquetball or squash you need the right protective eye wear.

There is no substitute for broadening personal knowledge of your chosen sport and to always choose the best equipment, especially when it relates to safety and well-being.

The same philosophy applies to technique. You should benefit from the accumulated experience of veterans who have distilled decades of trial and error to discover the most efficient and safe techniques applicable to a particular sport. Why should you retrace that path? Proper technique will ensure maximum enjoyment and maximum safety. Try wind-surfing without spending considerable time on proper technique and experience the excruciating frustration (to the point of anger and abandonment of the sport) flowing from unenlightened improvisation. Invest in your favorite sport.

(3) Slowly but Surely

The human body is slow in adapting to higher levels of exertion and, consequently, it needs a breaking-in period. This is a frequently neglected aspect of human physiology and is perhaps the most common reason for injuries. The rule of thumb is to increase the weekly intensity of exercise or its duration by 10%. One should then gradually attain a steady-state exercise level in 10 weeks. The jogging enthusiast should realistically expect to safely graduate from a sedentary lifestyle to running a 9-minute mile in three months.

The same principle applies after a lay-off. Unfortunately, one cannot bank the training effect. You lose your hard-earned exercise capacity rapidly - almost as rapidly as you gained it. After a few weeks of a lay-off, it is wise to resume the exercise routine with the same breaking-in parameters used originally. Slowly but surely you will regain your exercise proficiency.

Consistency is important. Don't be a week-end warrior, the local jock who sits in front of a computer all week and then thinks he can compete with Michael Jordan one-on-one or ace Pete Sampras for four straight hours on Saturday afternoon. You can't do it all in one day. You can't be sedentary all week and run a half-marathon on Sunday. The body dislikes inconsistency and is made vulnerable to injury by extreme bursts of activity. This is particularly true if there is heart disease or orthopedic fragility.

Moderation should rule. There is no known advantage in over-training. Unless you earn your living in a professional sport or the like, there is no good reason to go to extremes. It is not vital to run a marathon or swim across the English Channel. From a health point of view, there is no known benefit in going beyond a moderate level of exercise.

(4) Exercise Transitions

Just as you wouldn't charge your car out of the driveway on a cold winter morning, you shouldn't jump-start your exercise routine instantaneously. Approximately 10 minutes of warm-up exercises will ensure both the absence of injury and better performance. The warming-up process should include the muscles scheduled to bear the brunt of the exercise routine. Don't concentrate on warming up your shoulder muscles if you are planning to jog and vice-versa. I usually like to warm up by beginning with my regular work-out, but at a very reduced pace and then gradually increasing it over 8-10 minutes. For example, before a jogging stint, I like to walk slowly for two minutes, walk rapidly for two minutes, trot (15-minute mile) for an additional two minutes and then spontaneously merge into the steady-state intensity of an 8-9 minute mile.

This smooth breaking-in period is very effective and safe. Contrary to popular opinion, the warming-up period is not the right time for stretching exercises. They are not recommended for that purpose. Cold muscles, tendons and ligaments cannot be stretched adequately. It is strategically superior to save this activity for the cool-down period. Muscles are more amenable to stretching and less vulnerable to injury when warm.

A cool-down period is pleasant psychologically and advantageous physically. It lessens the incidence of muscle stiffness and hypotension (that could threaten the individual with heart or cerebrovascular disease). This is the perfect time to slowly "rev" down and enjoy the runner's high (a small compensation for all that hard work).

(5) Listen to your Body

If something doesn't feel right, it probably isn't. Pain is an indication of damage to tissues. This alarm bell should never be ignored. Either there is a flaw with the technique or there is overuse. Always listen to pain. Disregarding this simple signal is conducive to injury which, occasionally, will be serious and permanent. If you can't figure out what the problem is (wrong shoes, wrong technique, obesity, unnatural use or position, over-use) then seek professional help. Most often the problem is transparent. The poor battered body can't take the pounding and you should therefore pull back. If knee bends hurt your knees or shooting a jump shot hurts your back, it's time to abandon that activity and switch to another. There are so many syndromes related to the complications of exercise, from "tennis elbow" to "runner's toe" that one should refer to books on the subject or seek professional advice.

Adequate amounts of rest is the flip side of the exercise endeavour because so many complications are related to insufficient rest. It is helpful to visualize the sequence of events, as exercise causing micro-damage to working tissues which, subsequently, require enough time for the repair process. If the rate of damage regularly exceeds the rate of repair, dysfunction ensues. Adequate amounts of rest appropriate for the style and intensity of your personal exercise program is critically important.

One ploy to satisfy the demands of rest and repair, is to cross-train or alternate the types of exercises in order to use different muscle groups or different parts of the body on sequential days. This technique will protect against over-use, will diminish boredom and, finally, will assure a more comprehensive body conditioning.

(6) Be Security and Weather-Wise

Exercising outdoors requires special care. The temperature, direct sunlight, rain, snow, hail, lightning, humidity, wind, variable terrains and so on, must be considered. The outdoors environment is, in many ways, a minefield. Injury from tripping, twisting ankles, slipping, sunburn, frostbite, hypothermia, hyperthermia, dehydration, poor visibility, pollution, car accidents, dog attacks, getting lost - the list goes on - are all potential hazards. Common sense should prevail and the appropriate precautions taken. Keep identification on you, carry a bus ticket or money and don't go where the muggers go.

In the event of actual injury, apply the RICE principle:
- rest the injured area
- ice the area for about 20 minutes, allowing one hour between treatments; repeat frequently in the first 24-48 hours
- compress, through the application of an elastic tensor bandage
- elevate the injured area above the level of the heart
- do not "run through" an injury

The interface between the invigorating properties of a sound exercise program and chronic fatigue is problematic. Exercise is not indicated at all if fatigue is due to a medical condition, insufficient sleep or an overly-demanding workplace. In fact, under these circumstances, exercise may aggravate it. Exercise is particularly beneficial when a sedentary lifestyle has resulted in poor conditioning and inefficiency, when psychological problems dominate the landscape and, in most cases, when stress is at the root of the problem. The sedative properties of exercise are particularly helpful in the latter two.

Over-exercise is insidious. It does lead to chronic fatigue. The best way to substantiate the diagnosis is to temporarily suspend the exercise program and observe the results. Auspiciously, over-exercise is as rare as hen's teeth in our modern hedonistic culture.

NUTRITION

The ingestion of food to assemble the building blocks of organic life and to supply the life-sustaining energy fuels is so decisive in the struggle for survival that the evolutionary process has contrived powerful systems to compel it. Evolution has done so by conferring a survival advantage to species that developed irresistible appetites, wiley ruses to hunt effectively, superior stamina to travel long foraging distances, more efficient metabolisms and a more diversified diet. There is a clear-cut prejudice for food consumption and storage. The consequence is weaker control mechanisms to restrain the craving of food, its ingestion, its storage and its hormonal regulation.

What happens when food shortages are converted into food oversupply? The extraordinarily powerful instincts to consume run amok, poorly checked by weak natural control systems and lead to obesity. Obesity, ostensibly, is unhealthy, leading to countless adverse consequences in the human body. Table 10.5 summarizes the adverse health effects of obesity.

An intriguing bimodal phenomenon emerges: too little food will lead to energy depletion and fatigue directly, and too much food will lead to obesity, ill-health and fatigue indirectly.

TABLE 10.5
ADVERSE EFFECTS OF OBESITY

Blood lipids rise

Insulin resistance

Diabetes mellitus

Thyroid hormone decreases

Hypertension

Atherosclerosis

Coronary heart disease

Congestive heart failure

Peripheral vascular disease

Sleep-apnea syndrome

Snoring

Respiratory capacity is restricted

Respiratory failure

Degenerative arthritis

Injuries

Physical mobility diminishes

Peripheral venous disease

Risk of pulmonary embolism

Gallbladder stones

Physical beauty suffers

Negative image in society (low-class)

Reduces chances of professional success

Self-esteem crashes

Cost of living higher

Cancer rate increases

Happiness is spoiled

Mortality from cardiovascular disease increases

All cause mortality increases

Fatigue flourishes

Table 10.6 illustrates the health risks of an abnormal nutritional state. Too much or too little carries a heavy burden of organ dysfunction for entirely different reasons.

TABLE 10.6
NUTRITIONAL BALANCE

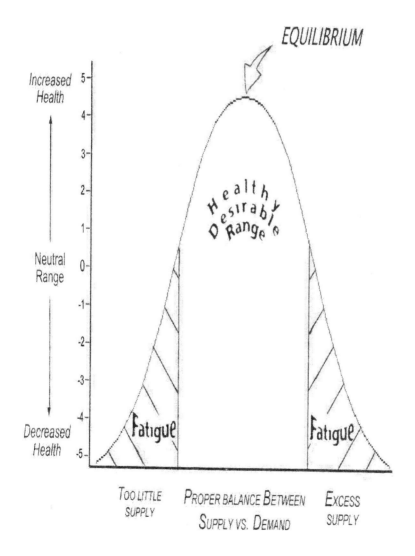

INADEQUATE NUTRITION

The prototypes are anorexia nervosa in the rich western societies and food scarcity in the Third World. Inadequate nutrition leads to weight loss, atrophy, weakness, innumerable pathological states and a dramatically lowered threshold for fatigue. The anorexic or bulimic victim is depleted of energy stores, has a malfunctioning metabolic system and, to top if off, risks serious illness up to sudden death from heart disease. Table 10.7 gives some examples of the consequences of a deficiency in essential nutrients.

TABLE 10.7
ADVERSE EFFECTS OF A DEFICIENCY
IN ESSENTIAL NUTRIENTS

Carbohydrates	Hypoglycemia
Fats	Hormonal deficiency
Protein	Malnutrition
Vitamin D	Rickets
Vitamin A	Night blindness
Vitamin E	Neuropathy
Vitamin K	Bleeding
Vitamin B_6 (pyridoxine)	Dermatitis
Vitamin C	Scurry
Nicotinic acid	Pellagra
Thiamine (B_1)	Encephalopathy
Iron	Anemia
Zinc	Dermatitis
Copper	Anemia
Manganese	Bleeding
Cobalt	Anemia
Chromium	Diabetes
Selenium	Cardiomyopathy
Fluoride	Bone loss
Calcium	Tetany
Magnesium	Confusion
Sodium	Seizures

| Potassium | Arrhythmias |
| Iodine | Hypothyroidism |

Note: For each deficiency, only one of many known clinical manifestations was selected, for the purpose of brevity.

The human body is similar to a giant factory where a whole assortment of primary and secondary products are necessary to produce its commodity. It needs fuels, lubricants, materials, electricity and the building blocks to manufacture the product. The human body requires a diversity of nutrients to sustain its many functions. Table 10.8 lists the essential dietary constituents of the human diet. Every single one of them is necessary for a healthful state.

Not only does the human body require its array of essential nutrients, it requires sufficient calories to meet its daily energetic requirements.

The calorie is a convenient measure of the amount of energy expended by the body and the amount of energy contained in a given foodstuff. One can then express supply and demand with one simple measure: the calorie.

The right amount of caloric supply (dietary intake) is pivotal for the integrity of the organism. Too little and the system degrades and too much, the body suffers the ill-effects of obesity.

An average healthy 45-year-old, 70 kg male who holds a sedentary job, requires approximately 2500 calories per day for his status quo. Of these 2500 calories, 1800 are for basal energy expenditure (basic requirements for operating the body), 500 for physical activity and 200 for nutritive expenditures (processing food).

TABLE 10.8
ESSENTIAL DIETARY CONSTITUENTS

ESSENTIAL	APPROXIMATE DAILY NUTRIENTS REQUIREMENT	
Carbohydrates (sugars)	—	
Lipids (fats)	—	
Essential fatty acids	1-2%	kcal
Proteins	45-65	g
Vitamin A	1000	ug
Vitamin D	5-10	mg
Vitamin E	10	mg
Vitamin K	45-80	ug
Vitamin C	50-60	mg
Thiamine	1.2-1.5	mg
Riboflavine	1.4-1.8	mg
Nicotinic acid	15-20	ug
Vitamin B$_6$	1.4-2	mg
Folates	150-200	ug
Vitamin B$_{12}$	2	ug
Biotin	30-100	ug
Pantothenic acid	4-10	mg
Calcium	800-1200	mg
Phosphorus	800-1200	mg
Magnesium	270-400	mg
Iron	10-12	mg
Zinc	15	mg
Iodine	150	ug
Selenium	40-70	ug
Copper	1.5-3	mg
Manganese	2-5	mg
Fluoride	1.5-4	mg
Chrome	50-200	ug
Molybdenium	75-250	ug

Daily caloric consumption must be adjusted upwards or downwards to gain weight, lose weight, compensate for illness, fever, stress, hormonal imbalance (overactive thyroid), amount of physical work, an exercise program and certain drugs. Each individual must fashion his or her diet to meet their own specific requirements. In problematic areas, self-education (there is no shortage of literature in this area) or the help from a professional in the field is indicated.

The fundamental message is simple: proper nutrition in terms of the appropriate numbers of calories consumed and the sufficiency of the broad range of essential nutrients is essential for optimal health. Optimal management of the energy supply-demand equation will ultimately dictate the threshold level for fatigue.

Fortunately, under-nutrition is rare in the prosperous West.

An interesting question that regularly surfaces in the context of fatigue is the value of over-consuming any of the essential nutrients. Is it beneficial for the chronic fatigue sufferer to consume more calories, more minerals and more vitamins than naturally required by the body? The short answer is no! There is no scientific evidence whatsoever to support the contention that, once functional requirements are satisfied, there is any benefit from over-consuming any of the essential nutrients. More on this in the final chapter.

EXCESSIVE NUTRITION AND OBESITY

Obesity has emerged as such a prevalent public health menace in many countries that it is rivaling cigarette smoking as a health concern. It is a veritable epidemic affecting approximately 33% of adults in the United States.

Obesity is defined as an excess of fat stored in adipose tissue. Body weight related to body surface area gives a rough estimate of the amount of adipose tissue in the body.

Classification of Obesity:

20 kg/m^2	=	underweight
$20\text{-}24.9 \text{ kg/m}^2$	=	ideal body weight
$25\text{-}29.9 \text{ kg/m}^2$	=	mild obesity
$30\text{-}40 \text{ kg/m}^2$	=	obesity
40 kg/m^2	=	severe obesity

Obesity will lower the threshold for fatigue or intensify it through:

- carrying excess weight, burdening any physical activity
- altering chest wall mechanics leading to an increased work of breathing
- increasing the work of the heart by expanding the circulation and by raising the blood pressure
- deconditioning is strongly associated with obesity - this lowers the threshold for fatigue
- the adverse medical consequences of obesity lead to fatigue indirectly - refer to Table 10.5 for a summary
- the negative psychological repercussions diminish self-esteem and contribute to depression, which is a direct cause of fatigue
- social, vocational or professional success is less likely and, consequently, curtails the boosting effect of these natural energizers
- sleep performance is often affected by the sleep-apnea syndrome (frequent in obesity)

The regulation of energy intake and expenditure is extraordinarily complicated. There are legions of hormones, neuro-peptides, kinins, prostaglandins and scores of neurological systems implicated in the web of signals and controls that will dictate human behavior. Suffice it to say that very little is known and success rates in combating obesity are abominably low.

This is not entirely surprising when one considers that evolution has favored the ingestion of food over restraining its intake. One may then enter a new aggregate of factors into the obesity equation:

seductive availability (of food)	+	diminished energy expenditure (technological explosion)	+	static control mechanisms (evolutionary basis)	=	Obesity

There is now a new evolutionary paradigm: "survival of the fittest" becomes "survival of the most disciplined".

TREATMENT OF OBESITY

Common obesity, in step with the false standard of ultra-thinness, is distributed on a Bell curve. There is such a thing as natural "plumpness", which is not particularly harmful from a health point-of-view. It is important to recognize it, as it is quite pointless to constantly fight nature. There are many set-points in human biology and weight is one of them. The first step is therefore to recognize when obesity is actually pathological.

The assessment of true pathological obesity is not straightforward, but it can be estimated reasonably well. Your weight history, your family history, your body morphology with a common sense juxtaposition against an analysis of energy intake (caloric consumption) versus energy expenditure (physical exertion) should result in some discernment of what is a reasonable weight for a given individual.

If a diagnosis of obesity is made, treatment is important. Unfortunately, medical science, at this point in time, knows just about everything about what doesn't work, and almost nothing about what does. Traditional dieting, cigarette smoking, stress, over-exercise, illness, intestinal bypass, gastroplasty, excess thyroid hormone, appetite suppressants (sympathomimetic drugs, serotonin-reuptake inhibitors) are either ineffective, too drastic or accompanied by unacceptable side-effects. Solution? There is none.

While there is no solution, the fundamental principles are still valid: total body weight is most influenced by the equilibrium between energy supply and demand. In other words, caloric intake must equate caloric expenditure to remain at any given body weight. The two critical variables are: dietary consumption and physical activity.

If you reduce caloric intake and increase your caloric expenditure with exercise you will lose weight and conquer obesity. The challenge is to institute these disciplines and sustain them.

Appetite suppresants investigated for the treatment of obesity include fluoxetine, a selective serotonin re-uptake inhibitor, fenfluramine and dexfenfluramine, which are serotonergic agents, and phenteramine and mazindol, which are noradrenergic agents. In most studies, there was a statistically significant difference in weight reduction during the initial phase of treatment in favor of the appetite suppressant group, but after this period, there was a general regaining of weight in all patient groups. Of much greater import, however, are the very serious side-effects reported with some of these drugs, notably pulmonary hypertension and cardiac valvular sclerosis (leading to valvular leakage).

Phentermine and fenfluramine (Phen-fen) have been removed from the market pending further studies.

Weight reduction surgery, gastric bypass, gastroplasty or intestinal bypass is indicated only for the most severe cases of morbid obesity.

Dietary counseling and behavioral therapy are, at best, modestly effective with typical early-phase success but later-phase slippage. Highly motivated people, however, appear capable of achieving sustainable weight loss. These fortunate individuals will reap the benefits flowing from their success: the opposite of all the known complications of obesity listed in Table 10.5 and improved fatiguability.

CHAPTER 11
WHEN FATIGUE HAS NO DOMINANT CAUSE

You are tired. Just plain tired. Can't seem to get going in the morning, work is agonizing, you drag your feet all day totally drained of any enthusiasm, you can't wait to hit the couch, vegetate and wither away life's precious moments dozing off in front of brain-dead TV programming. It seems that this state of affairs has been present forever with ups and downs. You consulted your doctor. All is normal. Laboratory tests are pristine. He has nothing to offer. You scratch your head trying to figure out what you are doing "wrong." You eat well, sleep well and exercise some. You are not overly stressed, at least not any more than your vigorous, bouncy and good-humoured friends, your workplace might not be exactly a playground but you cope, your boss is somewhat of a jerk but you can handle him, you don't smoke, drink, use drugs and party all night, so what's the problem?

Many people complain of chronic fatigue and no obvious cause is detectable. The group is highly heterogeneous. The largest sub-group is the ageing person (65 years of age and over) who does not realize that stamina progressively wanes with age. This is a simple fact of life. All bodily systems devitalize, become less effi-cient and, consequently, fatigue occurs more forcefully. Without this crucial knowledge, the maturing hyper-performing executive or housewife brutally crashes into the implacable wall of declin-ing energy stores and despairs. The insistence in maintaining the same lifestyle with declining capacity, will burden the unwitting victim with disabling fatigue.

The next largest subgroup is those who are constitutionally (genetically) designed with low energy levels. They are born tired and they die tired. We have all met them or we might be one ourselves. Seemingly, the physiological machinery and metabo-lism has low capacity. Fatigue therefore emerges ruthlessly when they attempt to perform at average levels of energy consumption. They clearly can't. If it is not possible to pare back activities to a level compatible with constitutional capabilities, chronic fatigue ensues.

A substantial number of people suffer from recurring fatigue because of global over-reaching where they stretch themselves to their outer limits in hundreds of little ways. The prototype might be a mother of two trying to advance a career and run a house-hold. Not a single factor stands out as responsible for fatigue but hundreds of little ones. There is a little too much hurrying, too much work, too little time, a bit too much stress, too little sleep or rest, not enough leisure time, unsatisfying sex, madcap eating habits, a few cigarettes here and there, a touch too much wine, harried vacations - in short, trying to hold 20 ounces of water in a 10-ounce glass. You get the picture. Chronic fatigue follows in-evitably.

Another group of fatigue sufferers with no dominant cause is represented by the individual who is generally unsatisfied with life. The unhappy person. You might call it a mild endogenous depression. Chronic dissatisfaction or unhappiness pervades the whole organism and robs it of the fires of life. The mechanism is unknown.

Another category of fatigue-sufferer is the medical patient afflicted with a debilitating illness which has no specific therapy. These patients suffer from chronic fatigue with a known cause, but a cause which cannot be eradicated. The approach to their fatigue will be the same as the others already alluded to. This group of people is afflicted with a grab-bag of diverse medical conditions. Examples are the Chronic Fatigue Syndrome, chronic viral illnesses such as hepatitis B or C and AIDS, chronic auto-immune disorders such as systemic lupus erythematosus (and other collagen-vascular diseases), degenerative neurological, or muscular diseases, such as multiple sclerosis and myopathies, chronic aplastic anemia, chronic pain of any kind, "fatiguing" medications that are nevertheless necessary for survival, and the list goes on.

Finally, there is idiopathic fatigue. A diagnosis by exclusion where no conceivable cause can be uncovered. An obsolete term from the 19th century describes it best: neurasthenia. Neurasthenics are always tired. They are most frequently female, young, somewhat tormented, have innumerable complaints including headaches, diffuse aches and pains (fibromyalgia), dizzy spells, numbness of hands and feet and are prone to hyperventilation. Their blood pressure is often very low, they are thin and pale. There is a high incidence of mitral valve prolapse (floppy mitral leaflets which can lead to leakage and cardiac irregularities), fibromyalgia, chronic fatigue syndrome, irritable bowel syndrome, dyspepsia (indigestion) and fainting spells. The outstanding feature, however, is profound fatiguability of body and mind. The underlying etiology of this tapestry of "functional" abnormalities is not known.

All these casualties of chronic fatigue can improve their lot immeasurably by following the simple, common sense approaches described in upcoming chapters. A major point must be made at the outset. There is no single, magical cure for fatigue. Its control requires multiple approaches with obsessive attention to every detail of living.

CHAPTER 12
THERAPY OF CHRONIC FATIGUE I:
ACHIEVE OPTIMAL PHYSICAL HEALTH

When a race car driving team is preparing for an important competition, they spend months modifying and fine-tuning the car to extract from it the best possible performance. No detail is overlooked. Every inch of the drive train, wheels, motor, is analyzed, perfected, re-tooled, until they have created a smooth-running masterpiece that will accomplish a most important assignment: win races. The more flawless the car, the better its performance and the more likely it will endure the challenge. Our physical make-up is not much different. The healthier, stronger and fitter every part of the body is, the better its function, efficiency and endurance. For somebody blessed with natural vivacity, this aspect of energy management is not so critical. For those with chronic fatigue, a well-oiled and perfectly-running piece of machinery is a cardinal rule. The first step in the battle against fatigue is to enhance the haleness of the body through and through.

An impeccably healthy lifestyle is crucial. The main compo-

Dr. Claude R. Maranda

nents follow:

HEALTHY NUTRITION

A well-balanced diet which contains all the essential nutrients (vitamins, minerals, fibers), the right proportion of carbohydrates (40% of calories), proteins (40% of calories), diversified fats (but mainly vegetable and fish oils) (20% of calories), and the correct number of total calories to maintain an ideal body weight. You can ignore the pseudoscientific hype of this whole field, the innumerable variants of dietary crafting, the power food of the year, the peculiar concoctions promising to boost your energy and all the hoopla surrounding natural products, megadose vitamins and assorted cure-alls. You can save a lot of time, grief and money if you just simply turn a deaf ear to all this blather. More on this in the last chapter.

Confirmed allergies to any foodstuff (e.g. gluten enteropathy) or intolerance (e.g. lactose intolerance) must be dealt with specifically.

TOP PHYSICAL CONDITIONING

Physical fitness is a profitable enterprise. It is, however double-edged. The victim of chronic fatigue carries a serious handicap: very little energy to sustain an exercise routine that will subsequently energize. The most reasonable way to handle this handicap is to ease oneself into a state of fitness more slowly, less intensely, more measuredly, more selectively, and customized to the needs and idiosyncracies of the individual. If a normal person can get into shape in three months, it might take the fatigue sufferer six months. Exercising mildly every second day may be all that can be negotiated. The key is to attempt the possible and achieve a minimum. If an exercise program seems counter-productive, aggravates fatigue and simply does not "feel right," abandon it and try something different. There is enough information in the popular literature to guide you in this important endeavor.

Instead of exercises designed for cardiopulmonary conditioning, the fatigue sufferer might benefit more from muscle toning and muscle strengthening exercises. Since most fatigue sufferers will lead relatively sedentary lifestyles they will rarely tap into excess cardiopulmonary capacity. However, stronger muscles will improve performance in everyday activities and as such will pay more dividends. It is also fateful that a stronger muscle has a higher threshold for fatigue. An added bonus.

Exercise has many other benefits for the fatigue sufferer. It is good preventive medicine for cardiovascular illness and osteoporosis, both of which could theoretically add to the overall burden of debility. Furthermore, exercise enhances the quality of sleep and it has a natural anti-depressant effect both of which are invaluable in this context.

PLENTIFUL REST

Whatever it takes, do it. It is axiomatic that there must be an equilibrium between work and rest. If nine to ten hours of sleep with a sprinkling of daytime naps are what it takes to make life tolerable, it would be rather masochistic not to abide by nature's imperatives.

Napping must be dedicated. The attention to the same details applicable to sleep in Chapter 10 is in order. To be recuperative, a nap must be focused on just that. Watching TV, reading a book, meditating, listening to music and attempting to nap in an uncomfortable position just won't cut it. These activities sustain alertness, which is antithetic to restorative rest. This type of rest (as opposed to resting a muscle) is a central nervous system rehabilitation so the brain must shut off.

Napping in the workplace is not looked upon favorably and, mistakenly, it is perceived as laziness or an indicator of a wild lifestyle. This is unfortunate because even perfectly healthy people gain in productivity when critical napping is instituted. The fatigue sufferer should use coffee breaks and the lunch hour to find a quiet spot and nap. If he happens to have an enlightened boss, more effective measures can be arranged.

PREVENTIVE MEDICINE

Preventive medicine is an integral part of a strategy to maintain top physical health through a lifetime. Chronic fatigue sufferers cannot afford to degrade in any way their capital of energy. So, to the extent you can avoid preventable illnesses, your lifetime battle position is enhanced.

Simple measures to introduce:

- institute all safety measures to prevent motor vehicle and motorcycle mishaps (seat belts, avoid cell phones, wear helmets etc).
- be aware of and avoid pedestrian accidents (avoiding high volume and high speed crossings, sports playing on streets)
- wearing safety equipment for any sport (e.g. helmets when bicycling)
- accident-proof your house and workplace (sharp corners, low-lying objects for head injuries, slippery mats, high water temperature)
- dispose of all potentially toxic chemicals
- smoke detectors and abiding by inflammable standards for sleep-ware
- pool security and swimming precautions
- eliminate firearms
- assiduous control of coronary risk factors which put you at risk for the high morbidity and mortality of vascular atherosclerosis: smoking, high cholesterol, obesity, sedentary lifestyle, diabetes mellitus, hypertension being the main ones. Your physician will be an invaluable source of information for optimal management.
- Cancer screening
Breast self-examination and mammography, prostate exam

and measurement of the prostate-specific antigen, fecal occult blood examination and sigmoidoscopy for colorectal cancer, Pap smears for cervical cancer, genetic screening when there is a strong family history.

- Cigarette smoking cessation is an absolute must: the massive amount of data accumulated on the harmful effects of cigarette smoking should provide a powerful motivational environment. That, plus ingenious new methods to help the quitting process (support groups, nicotine replacement therapy by a variety of routes and Bupropion (Zyban) arm the addict with effective tools to kick the habit).
- Potentially noxious respiratory inhalants should be avoided: fumes, dusts, allergens. The flu vaccine and the Pneumovax (vaccine against pneumococcal pneumonia) are indicated in high-risk individuals (the elderly and the immune-deficient).
- Hepatitis B immunization
- any substance abuse should be eradicated
- avoid exposure to infectious agents: no contact whatsoever with infected individuals, protected sex, avoidance of endemic areas (if not possible, use prophylactic antibiotics), meticulous hygiene, sound cooking practices
- Annual medical check-up: a periodic health examination might not be cost-effective in a healthy population. However, chronic fatigue sufferers, by virtue of their diminished resistance to illness and their greater susceptibility to any form of debilitating process, will benefit from frequent medical evaluation and guidance.

CHAPTER 13
THERAPY OF CHRONIC FATIGUE II:
ENHANCE PSYCHOLOGICAL WELL-BEING

An obviously important component of the overall strategy to combat fatigue is to enter the battlefield with maximum psychological health and resistance. This aspect of the mission is so critical that a major effort must be expended in this area. The point cannot be over-emphasized. The psychological climate is pre-eminent.

Psychological well-being is not a wayward state like the untethered sails of a boat twisting and turning in the winds of positive and negative emotions. It is a fundamental, biological quantity that has played a pivotal role in the evolution of the animal species. Emotions do not exist just for whim. They have a mission to guide, protect and propel the animal in the path that best ensures its most important goals on earth: to survive, to reproduce and to thrive. There is an unbreakable link between psychological well-being and the success in fulfilling those three biological mandates. The more a person assures his survival, the more reproduction is facilitated and the more a person thrives physically, socially and morally, the greater the psychological well-being. It is inextricably rooted in pure biology.

In practical terms, the key constituents of psychological well-being are security (survival), self-esteem (thriving), love (reproduction) and a fourth one, realistic expectations.

SECURITY

Security is an all-encompassing hallmark of the struggle to survive. Consider the complete absence of security, financial, physical and social (for example, bankruptcy, an oppressed minority in the grip of a civil war, a homeless person) and you will readily acknowledge that happiness and serenity would be virtually impossible. The stronger you are, the richer you are, the more access you have to resources, and the broader your support network, the more security you enjoy. The mission is therefore straightforward. Build a cushion of security as thick as you can muster. This implies a good job, an adequate income, a good neighborhood, a strong family base, good friends, and an intelligent avoidance of the common risks inherent in society, especially the risk of violent crimes. How does one achieve this? Knowledge, hard work, intelligence, image and luck.

SELF-ESTEEM

Self-esteem is how we view ourselves. It is a product of reflective consciousness appraising our worth: worth to ourselves, our loved ones and society in general. This determination of worth is mostly subjective and susceptible to the many perceptual distortions inherent to the human mind. Low self-esteem, then, could result from an inaccurate assessment of oneself or may be right on the mark, if one is a failure. Both must be rectified.

Low self-esteem does not *per se* worsen fatigue. It does so, however, indirectly, by influencing the many aspects of life that impact on the state of fatigue. If we look at the negative consequences of low self-esteem, one will understand why.

Consequences of low self-esteem:

- feelings of inadequacy, incompetence and impotence leading to a state of functional paralysis
- conflicting feelings for loved ones
- sensitivity to rejection
- compulsion to punish or be punished
- social isolation, shyness
- strong urges to control and manipulate
- depression and anxiety
- lost opportunities, waste of time (hesitation)
- high risk for substance abuse
- lack of self-acceptance
- sexual dysfunction
- self-defeating behavior and crime
- fear of intimacy and of success
- underachievement
- spouse battering or child molestation
- inappropriate pregnancies and failed marriages
- suicide and crimes of violence
- One can readily see the poisonous attributes of low self-esteem and how it might act as a major magnifier of fatigue. How to enhance self-esteem? The following suggestions should be helpful.

(1) Know Thyself and Accept Thyself

Self-knowledge is a universal principle espoused by all serious students of human nature. This is the first step in aligning the capabilities of the self and reality. Without the knowledge of the strengths and weaknesses, the natural talents, likes and dislikes and the temperamental tolerance levels of the psycho-biological fiber of the self, there will inevitably be mismatching between what is desired and what is possible. Mismatching breeds stress and loss of self-esteem. How could one properly establish self-esteem if life's agitations are constantly in a state of dysequilibrium? Not possible. Perceptive self-knowledge, enlightened life choices, in tune with that knowledge, will breed wisdom and, with the same delivery, self-acceptance. The latter is an elementary product of a clear understanding of the nature of man and humility.

(2) Know your Environment

To assess your performance and to judge the success of your efforts, you must know and understand your environment. You have to evaluate, realistically, what is possible, what is fantasy, a waste of time, a good opportunity, favorable conditions and so on. General knowledge of sociology, business, politics, law, psychology, basic sciences and philosophy is, by far, the best conveyor of the needed perspective to make intelligent choices. What your visions are, what your goals should be, in short, what your destiny on earth is, depends on the proper matching of your capabilities with the opportunities offered by your environment. Only within this context can you nourish self-esteem.

(3) Live Responsibly and Authentically

Choices in life, from the peccadillo to life-altering decisions, rests entirely on your shoulders. No one else is responsible. There must be full respect for reality, knowledge and truth. Appropriate choices will foster the sense of serenity that comes with responsible decisions.

Authentic living is a derivative of responsible living. There is no gain in living a lie. Much energy, time and self-esteem is wasted on projecting attitudes and images that do not reflect your true inner self. This mode of behavior is self-defeating. The conflict arising from incongruent inner and external lives will destroy you. One must muster the courage to project who and what he is. The converse is a virtual rejection of oneself with its attendant depressing effects on self-esteem.

(4) Cultivate Positive Attitudes

Attitudes are malleable with self-discipline and perseverance. Neural plasticity allows for modification of long-established neural networks. Plasticity is a neurological learning mechanism where nerve cells either re-connect themselves differently or increase the density of couplings between them, creating a richer communication network .Repetition and intensity (like physical exercise) will gradually reshape attitudinal leanings through plasticity.

- Choose activism over passivism. Why let events control you when it is in your power to influence them?
- Choose assertiveness over submission. You are as good and legitimate as anybody else. Why take a back seat? If you know your capabilities and your limits, press ahead with your responsible choices.
- Choose confidence over shyness. Shyness is conquerable by desensitization (repeated exposure), physical relaxation techniques, humor, practice, self-talk, optimism, abandonment of perfectionism, regression of self-deprecatory reflexes, allowance for rejection, searching for comfort zones, and not accepting worst-case scenarios.
- Choose benevolence over self-centredness. The theory affirms that the returns are larger than the investment.
- Choose optimism over pessimism. Optimism costs nothing. It provides the motivating fuel for action. Why not nurture it?

(5) Dismantle Negative Attitudes

Regardless of the pathophysiology of negative attitudes, be they the product of a loveless and neglected youth or a genetically-determined temperamental bias, they can be eradicated.

Negative thoughts, from feelings of guilt to incompetence, should be recognized. Once recognized, they should be systematically defined as to their triggers, settings and underlying reasons. Repress them. Be alert to their very incipience, catch yourself in the act and pulverize them. Self-deprecatory reflexes can be disarmed. Re-interpret the conditions that regularly trigger these thoughts. Slowly but surely, you will win the tussle.

(6) Search for Excellence

Since most of our self-esteem is based on how valuable a human being we actually are, any effort to upgrade that raw capital will proportionately enhance it (self-esteem). Every step towards excellence in any segment of our being, necessarily has an uplifting effect. The heart of the strategy is to upgrade as much as is humanly possible every single aspect of our existence:

- health and beauty
- intelligence and knowledge
- emotional stability
- social skills
- professional and financial achievements
- love
- altruism and moral eminence

(7) Love

When you love someone, that person becomes very important, very significant to you. The flip side, to be loved, is to be made important and of great value to someone else. This enhancement of value feeds your self-esteem. Love is a very powerful component of self-esteem. When you are loved, it makes you feel attractive, good, successful and, most of all, significant.

At the end of the line, the more love you inject into your life, be it romantic, family, religious or social, the more your self-esteem rises.

Sources of love are plentiful and opportunities abound for anybody who cares to look for them:

- girlfriends, boyfriends or spouse (not simultaneously!)
- immediate family
- extended family, distant relatives
- friends, neighbors, acquaintances
- workmates, clubs, institutions
- society at large, altruism
- God
- pets (especially dogs!)

(8) Religion

Religious conviction confers a *de facto* enrichment of self-esteem. You are of high value because you are created in the image of God and he loves you more completely and more perfectly than any love found on earth. When your life is in harmony with the Will of God, high self-esteem is a non-issue: it is intrinsic.

(9) A Unique Skill

Any unique skill or achievement, however banal it might seem to outsiders, will boost self-esteem because you are the best at something. That something is not nearly as important as the fact that you are the best. Obviously being the best tennis player in the world is a more potent ego-booster than, say, beer-bottle collecting. Nevertheless, symbolism plays an enormous role. You need not be a recipient of the Nobel prize, nor be a movie star. All you need is your own personal conviction that there is something in your life you feel you do very well. If it's a trick on your bicycle, staying under water for two minutes, dunking a basketball, carving a sling-shot, drawing pictures, collecting bugs, playing a musical instrument, a special hair style, a beer chug-a-lugging winner, and so on, it's enough to validate you. Evaluate your own natural talents or your personal interests and find your own specialty. If it also happens to be socially redeeming or useful or even lucrative, so much the better. But these attributes are not prerequisites.

One caveat. Stay away from competitive activities like chess or adversarial sports. Too few are winners. The chances of you being the best are minuscule. There is always someone smarter or stronger than you are. What is the point of subjecting yourself to ego-battering competitive activities on a regular basis? Not an intelligent way of boosting your self-esteem.

(10) Altruism

A pure gift to humanity, no strings attached, is an invaluable enhancer of self-esteem. Any form of untethered generosity towards society, such as volunteering or charity work, civic deeds, social work of any type, does two things for you: it makes you valuable to society and it tells you that you are a good person. What better way to shore up your self-esteem? Find a hospital, a food bank, a preservation society, an amateur sporting activity, a school program etc., and give of yourself. The benefits you will reap are incalculable.

LOVE

Love is the third pillar of psychological well-being. In fact, without it, no animal life (including us) would exist on earth. Love is the attraction between two organisms for the purpose of reproduction. This is as true for a unicellular organism as it is for the most highly evolved animal on the planet, *Homo sapiens*. This mysterious impulse urges reproduction, fosters a will to nurture and protect the offspring, and consolidates any position that promotes the well-being of that progeny. The more direct the link between the reproductive arena and any other factor in life, the more powerful will be the sensation of love. For example, the most powerful loves are the love of self, mate and child as they are directly implicated in the imperative to reproduce. Loves for money, friends, God and country are not as powerful as their nexus with the production and protection of progeny is weaker and indirect. Table 13.1 presents a conceptualized graph of the relationship of the intensity of love with the proximity to genetic reproduction.

Because love is a primary, irrepressible and essential element of humanity, its fulfilment will have a major impact on general psychological well-being. The more love there is in one's life (loves of all kinds) the better the psychological climate. This, in turn, will influence the threshold for fatigue.

Strategies to enrich our lives with love, particularly the most precious ones, romantic and reproductive love, are plentiful.

TABLE 13.1
THE POWER OF LOVE

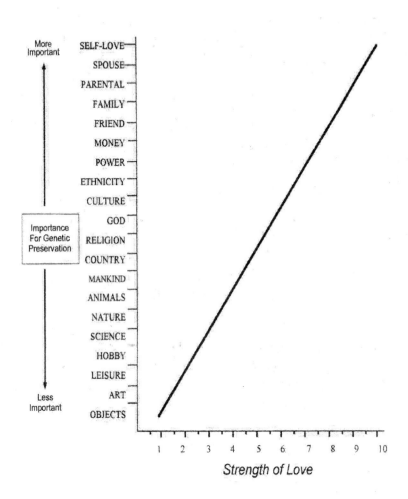

Strength of Love

ROMANTIC AND REPRODUCTIVE LOVE

Reproduction is so crucial for the survival of living organisms that nature imparted to this endeavor its most exquisite rewards. The ultimate human ecstasies are those attached to romantic love and the ultimate physical pleasure is that of the sexual orgasm. It represents the confirmation of a successful consummation of the mating ritual. No other pleasure in life can stoke the fires of pure raw desire as those can. They can literally drive a human being insane. No wonder the appropriate management of this super-heated component of life is so complex, delicate and full of pit-falls.

(1)   Square Your Dreams with Reality

Love is so enthralling, and sexual desire so powerful, that they both overwhelm reality and distort it. The phenomenon of per-ceptual diffraction and blurring associated with love is very sim-ply nature's way of overcoming the gruesome banality of life. Anything to favor reproduction. The danger for the unsuspecting love-struck paramour is the misinterpretation of the inevitable reality check that follows. Better be prepared than get ambushed by unnecessary painful misunderstandings.

The most common distorted perceptions of love are:

- The belief that intense passionate love will endure the test of time, never wane and last a lifetime. Absolutely not. Erotic love and its variants typically accedes its peak very early in a relationship (weeks) and wanes to approximately half-intensity in six to eighteen months. Presumably the phenomenon of desensitization (down-regulation of re-ceptors or tolerance) is responsible for this. No need to panic! This is perfectly physiological. One should not in-terpret this natural decrement in passion as a diminish-ment of love. It is simply an evolutionary step in a com-plex human relationship.
- The belief that the loved one is unique, exceptional, the most beautiful person on earth and other assorted unreal-

148

istic attributes limited only by the over-stimulated imagination of the lover. Don't kid yourself. Your loved one is not unique, exceptional or the most anything: you only think he or she is. Love is indulging your brain. As the passion wanes, you will gradually realize that your little love bud and treasure is no different than that plain Jane next door or your friend's wife. It is just a matter of time. Again, it is better to understand this sooner rather than later.

- The belief that your whole life's happiness depends on that singular loved one. This is rarely actually the case. There are many fish in the sea. If you miss out on one, there is most assuredly another one equally as alluring just around the reef.
- The belief that life with the loved one is a guarantee of blissful serenity. This is a no-brainer. Conflict is inevitable. Conflict is inherent to the mating game, as men and women have evolved quite different strategies to solve mating problems. Men are more driven by the copulative aspects of mating, are more aggressive, less discriminatory in their choice of mate particularly for casual sex for which they have a great predilection, are less attuned to the nurturing aspects of love and are less sympathetic to the concepts of commitment, fidelity and altruism. Women, on the other hand, are completely different. Sex *per se* is less critical; they are more passive, infinitely more choosy as to the choice of a prospective mate, are not subject to agreeing to casual sex so readily as the consequences of a full pregnancy and the responsibilities of nurturing the offspring makes them very reluctant to gamble; are much more inclined to emphasize the nurturing aspects of love and thrive on the realization of commitment, devotion and fidelity. These distinct differences in the partners of the love game provide a fertile soil for innumerable types of conflicts. The extrapolation here is that, when engaging in a loving

relationship, an alertness to the tremendous potential for conflict and the understanding of the evolutionary basis of these conflicts arms the paramour with the necessary tools for success.

- The belief that your love interest is inevitably attracted to you. This delusion is more prevalent in men. How can women resist this incredible hunk that I am? Unfortunately, very easily.

- The belief that the grass is greener on the other side of the fence. It isn't. The insatiable quest for better or sexier is almost always rewarded with disappointment. Once you have fallen in love with a significant other, it is very unlikely that comparison-shopping for the ultimate love, will ever bring you happiness. The more things change, the more they remain the same. Keep your reliable old Ford! The glitzy European sports car is probably a barrelful of headaches.

- The belief that love and sexual drive are easy to control. Love and sex are highly addictive. Just as addictive as heroin and cocaine. Not surprising, as the same neurons and neurotransmitters underlie their beguiling effect. If you are genetically predisposed to addiction (check your family history), if you know you harbor an addictive personality or if you are already in the grips of a love or sex addiction, then specific action is in order. The potential for life-wrecking mishaps is just as great, if not greater, as with heroin, cocaine or alcohol addiction. While there is no known cure, preventive or palliative measures exist to help remedy the situation. These measures closely parallel the ones generally used for drug addiction (unfortunately not enough).

- Make Yourself Attractive
  Beauty is magnetic. Physical appearance is the very first criterion that will initially classify you as a potential love mate or not. It is not the definitive one, but is often the

initial spark that triggers the conflagration. This initial critical step is advantaged by "beautification." By simple attention to detail, and at almost no cost to you, you can enhance your physical appeal no matter what your starting point is. Physical beauty, by implying good health and quality genes, will make you a more attractive love prospect. While males place a higher premium on female beauty, one should not be surprised that male beauty is also a significant factor in the female decision tree (simply consider the startling fact that our ancestral progenitors assigned the burden of displaying physical beauty on the shoulders of the male).

Just as important as physical beauty is inner beauty. You sense it. It is a product of basic happiness, health, confidence, optimism, strength and serenity. Inner beauty is a cue for success. Success is a cue for quality. Quality makes you more desirable. A simple technique to exude inner beauty: smile, always smile, never not smile. There is no other single, most effective expression of inner beauty than the human smile. Smile all the time and you will be amazed at how people will gravitate towards you. Smile. It's magical!

(3)   Strive for Excellence

Have you ever wondered why the football star gets all the girls or a famous (or powerful) person attracts the opposite sex like "bees to honey"? There is no aphrodisiac like success: excellence in sports, the performing arts, science, art, business, politics, religion and literature, most of which can be indirectly measured by the great barometers of wealth and power, are extremely potent generators of romantic attraction. Why? Because they reflect promising genes and therefore make you a most desirable mate. As simple as that. The evolutionary tractor has crushed any other competing strategy.

Success, which is an indirect estimate of genetic fitness, need not be absolute! There is no possibility that the vast majority of us poor earthlings will ever achieve success on a grand scale. Of course not! It's all relative. Within our own small universe, we can strive for relative success in anything and achieve the same result. It boils down to excellence. The more you cultivate a high degree of excellence and in as many aspects of your life as possible, the more successful your romantic ventures will be.

Excellence in image, physical prowess, intelligence, knowledge, skills, profession and/or social status; in short, excellence, through and through, will proportionately enhance your chances of fashioning a satisfactory love life. Proof? We are the proof. We are the product of an evolutionary process where the excellent win, survive and reproduce and the less excellent disappear (at least their genes do).

(4)   Nurture the Qualities that Promote Love

Have you ever asked yourself this question: "What are the decisive human qualities that unconsciously drive the selection of a love mate?" The answer lies in the fundamental prerequisites of human coupling that have enabled reproduction and nurturing of the offspring. For the male, the attributes are the capacity to provide resources (economic capacity) and all its appurtenances, in addition to commitment as reflected by devotion, kindness and fidelity. For females, the attributes are youth, fertility and devotion (nurturing). These evolution-inspired insights conjure us to nourish these qualities for the optimization of loving relationships.

Mating strategies are deeply rooted in our ancestral history. We are the product of evolutionary struggles with their successes and failures. The female of the species has emerged as a well-honed detector of the qualities in a male that will best ensure the survival of her offspring. Commitment emerges as a key constituent. The more resources a male will commit to the relationship, the better. The capacity to provide food, shelter and security, is highly prized. A high social status, with its greater access to resources (power, prestige, privilege), dependability, which reduces the threat of withdrawal of resources, fidelity, which reassures the female that the male's resources will not be squandered on other females, are all attributes that a woman will take into consideration when choosing a mate.

Ambition and industriousness are powerful predictors of future income and professional accomplishment. They are extremely important qualities as they reveal the likelihood that the prospective partner is a promising one. Lack of ambition and laziness are extremely undesirable traits and, consequently, spoil any chance of attracting a good mate.

(5) Perfect Health Makes Perfect Love

A healthy person beams. His/her physical appearance is resplendent, his/her mood up-beat, he/she displays high energy and his/her body language exudes rhythm and sensuality. Good health makes a person alluring. The converse is a significant deterrent to mating. Our ancestors recognized that ill-health conferred a risk of contamination, a clue to incompetence, a risk of dying prematurely (before the offspring reaches independence), and a signal of low-quality genes. Nature is not kind to the unhealthy.

(6) Train Your Intelligence

While your native I.Q. is likely primarily genetically-determined, there is ample room for improving your practical intelligence, your emotional intelligence, your social skills and your fund of knowledge to develop a resplendent image of intelligence. Speech training, formal and informal education, mental gymnastics, the aggressive accumulation of knowledge and the flourishing of wisdom by learning from the best, will all contribute to your overall intelligence. Why? Because intelligence is a potent predictor of prosperity. The higher you rate, the more attractive a mate you will be.

(7) Be Available

There is ample love out there waiting for you. You have to find it and it has to find you. No amount of head-bashing will compensate for an isolationist attitude. Like the random Brownian motion of particles in fluid, you need to circulate, contact as many people as possible and immerse yourself in a sea of "connective" opportunity. The more you expose yourself to the swarms of humanity, the more likely you are to find a pearl. You must analyze your environment (availability of social contacts) and focus all your efforts on facilitating and multiplying human contacts. This is facilitated by frequenting schools, libraries, clubs, parks, cruises, parades, dog-walking, volunteer work, cafeterias, beaches, churches, sports (or other events). Just let your imagination take over. There are countless ways of increasing the number of human interactions. You have to "go out there" and "display yourself." Eventually, a golden opportunity will turn up.

(8) Be Receptive

You might not be the most beautiful, sexy or intelligent person on earth but you certainly can transform yourself into a warm, welcoming, pleasant, non-threatening and most comfortable human being. People will flock to you. Friends will cherish you. Your spouse will not resent waning passion and will treasure the simple, comfortable and warm companionship that you provide.

(9) Pet Love

The phenomenon of unconditional pet-owner love is intriguing. Why is it that pet owners feel so much love for their pets, a love that is fierce and unfettered, without waning or spoiling. The bond between the pet and its master is unseverable and certainly endures more than most marriages. If we could extract and package this secret ingredient of the pet-human bond, this incredible love, it would break all retailing records hands down!

What makes this love so deep, so sincere and so durable? Nobody knows. One would suspect that many factors come into play:

- unconditional affection
- predictability
- attentiveness
- untethered
- always appreciative
- non-threatening
- vulnerable, appeals to nurturing instincts
- companionship
- makes you feel important thereby increasing self-esteem
- no intellectualization, no arguments

- provides a refuge from stress
- security
- loyalty

The factors responsible for this phenomenon should be incorporated in your play book for the grand game of love. It is highly likely that the pet phenomenon, the combination of secure, attentive, patient, undemanding, non-threatening and unconditional love with the qualities of true friendship and companionship, is a profitable course to follow. It certainly works for dogs. Need we be so different from our immediate ancestors?

(10) Sexual Adequacy

The actual performance of the sexual act is much more than the mere copulative union of two sexual partners breathlessly reaching an orgasmic climax. There is a whole aura of epiphenomena and symbolism surrounding sex which fully transcends the actual physical act. The physiologic and psychological repercussions of mating are momentous. Adequate, competent and confident sexual performance has a direct impact on love, its full expression and its endurance. You cannot dissociate love and sex because they are the natural link of reproduction. The first cracks in a love relationship are first seen in the sexual arena and the first sign of sexual indifference has a direct impact on the quality and quantity of love. Symbolism runs deep.

The message is straightforward. Be as competent and loving a sexual partner as possible in the full natural sense of the words. Any real, suspected or perceived problem has a remedy and it should be applied.

(11) Listen to Your Heart

Reproduction has been around for approximately three billion years and serious intellectual development, perhaps several hundred thousand years. If you had to choose, which one would you rely on for inspiration. To put the issue in context, consider this. Reproduction has successfully managed life for three billion years with a track record of engineering a measly string of amino acids into a masterpiece which is man. On the other hand, our great intellects have spawned the most bizarre, flawed, conflicting, contradictory and confused political systems, legal systems and religious systems which makes you wonder about the computing quality of our central nervous system. I believe that nature's track record is a testimony to its superior ability as a guide for behavior. Our intellectual faculties should be restrained to researching why nature works so well.

Therefore, trust your instincts, your deep emotion-laden subliminal biological impulses. More times than not, these impulses point in the right direction. There is a fundamental reason for every feeling, impulse, appetite and the reason is usually biological and usually on the mark. Your "love instinct" has been finely-honed for several billion years. It should be your best guide.

How do you distinguish valid biological impulses or instincts from aberrant or distorted ones? Time will tell. The generation of happiness will be the indication. If your line of action generates a sense of genuine happiness, it is likely to be correct. If the result is an uneasy sense of unhappiness, something is usually wrong. Change your strategy accordingly.

(12) Compatibility Reduces Fallibility

There is a sense that love is more natural and spontaneous between people who are alike rather than dissimilar. Experience supports the contention that love is more enduring between people of similar race, religion, culture, politics, social class, intellectual level, interests and lifestyles. It is tempting to accept the thesis that too much dissimilarity is bound to be associated with a heavy burden of conflict. True. But on the other hand, too much similarity implies too much genetic similarity. This presents evolutionary dangers to the species. Probably the middle of the road is what nature would advise. Phenotypic (physical) similarity is probably not a biologically favorable basis for attraction (genetically too close), but temperamental or psychological similarities probably provide a more fertile soil for love, endurant love.

With that perspective in mind, one should attempt to meet potential mates with similar inclinations. In other words, if you are a rock-a-billy construction worker whose pleasurable climax in life is to watch wrestling on TV with a twelve-pack, don't take fine arts courses at the local school. You are not likely to find a convivial mate there.

Successful long-term relationships require a sustained cooperative alliance. Studies show that the more dissimilarities there are in a married couple, the greater the divorce rate. Good psycho-social matching is therefore an important consideration. Similarities of race, culture, intelligence, education, social class, religious beliefs, political beliefs and visions will reduce the frequency and intensity of conflicts. Mutually incompatible goals are very costly in a relationship and will often lead to its ruination.

(13) Give Love and You Will Receive Love

This attitude of the heart is a most profitable one. By showering love genuinely and without strings attached, it will be returned two-fold. This is not a paradox. Love breeds love. There is an apparent risk involved, however. You are not guaranteed love in return but the probabilities are high. One should fearlessly plunge forward on that route: the rewards are immense. Mother nature has made it quite clear. If you are sincere, benign and an asset to another individual, that other person will be attracted to you, will search for you, will yearn for you and will love you. It's one of those little pearls of love.

REALISM

The fourth pillar of psychological well-being is realism. Realism is an accurate gauging of reality coupled with commonsense. The converse is fantasy, magical thinking and delusions. While the latter might provide short-term gain, a day of reckoning awaits around the corner. There is no conceivable advantage in daydreaming through life, wearing rose-colored glasses and "imagining" unworkable schemes. Why? Because a lion's share of our psychological well-being rests on how our performance in life matches our expectations. If one is riding high on lofty expectations and never quite attains them, there will result debilitating dissatisfaction. Setting goals that are out of reach is a recipe for unhappiness; there is an emotional price to pay: mal-contentment, cynicism, depression, exasperation - all powerful generators of fatigue.

An important aspect of realism is the interplay of expectations with reality in the realm of people comparisons. We all do it. We compare ourselves in looks, size (height, muscles), prowess, occupation, beauty of spouse, intelligence of children, size and price of the home, wealth, cars etc. You name it and we compare it. Much of our state of mind depends on how we measure up to "the competition." The problem is two-fold: there is always "bigger and better" and most comparisons are not valid. Each human being is unique, different, flawed in many ways and the whole panorama of qualities and characters is beyond simple comparisons. So why bother? True, the observation of excellence and success stories is inspiring and can spur one to great things. This is fine if the quest is realistic. It boils down to the basic tenet that one should accurately evaluate one's potential and strive for what is possible. To do otherwise is a high-risk venture: a debilitating waste of energy based on an unthinking line of action that has almost no chance of being fruitful. There are better ways of proceeding. We would all be further ahead by leaving fantasy to Hollywood.

A state of healthy realism can only be achieved with knowledge - knowledge of oneself and knowledge of the world we live in.

CHAPTER 14
THERAPY OF CHRONIC FATIGUE III:
UPGRADE YOUR POSITION IN SOCIETY

We are social animals and we are interdependent. The chronic fatigue sufferer will need to search out the most comfortable and secure position in this complex and perilous community. Complex is self-evident. Perilous, not only because of possible violence but because the constant interaction between members of a society provides a rich environment for stress, conflict and debasement. Marriage, the workplace, the public arena are sources of extraordinary gratification but are also double-edged: they can be a ruinous drain of the limited energetic resources of the victim of chronic fatigue.

The management of societal life is an art. Experience is invaluable. A solid knowledge of human nature is indispensable. It takes many decades to succeed. Certain broad principles should be understood early in the ball game.

- Society is both a cooperative union and an intensely competitive one. One must walk a fine line between them. Too much of either is risky. Too much cooperation can lead to exploitation and too aggressive a competitive stand creates dangerous enemies. Each one of us must discover this fine line. No formula will apply to everybody.

- Conformity is cherished. Have you ever noticed how much mimicry there is in human relations? Customs, mores, mannerisms, accents, fashions, culture, are all manifestations of this phenomenon of mimicry. It has always astounded me how often a patient, sitting across my desk will adopt postures and hand positions that mirror mine. I have tested this phenomenon on many occasions. If you cross your arms, cock your head, lean your face on a hand, scratch your head, join your hands etc. etc., you can observe the unsuspecting person mimic the same motions or positions. Laughing is infectious, yawning is contagious, speech patterns are mimicked and the list is endless. This quirk of human nature is an important clue to successful behavior in society. Mimicry is equal to conformity. Conformity equals joining forces and cooperation. This translates into friendship, benignity and an expansion of security. Society loves conformity. Nothing stimulates conflict, hatred and overt racism more than "being different." Difference in color, language, race, culture, religion, politics and social status can be a marker for societal discrimination and attack. The message is not that one can change human nature. That cannot be done (except over many centuries if not millennia). The message is that, at a practical level, one should strive to blend in fully with the prevailing culture so as not to stand out as a sore thumb. If your mission in life is to shock, be an eccentric and a trail-blazer, fine; arm yourself accordingly. If, on the other hand, you are a fatigue sufferer, you can't afford the high cost. Play by the unwritten rules. Conformity is the essence of harmony.
- Use the power of social candy. Need or want to get something done? Forget coercion, fear or bullying. The short-

term gain is not worth the long-term pain. Use candy. Incentives are infinitely more effective. If you want to be successful in society, play this card to its maximum.

- Recognize what motivates people. The fundamental motivations of the human animal are biological. They are certainly not religious. If they were, there would be no wars, no crime and no stress to speak of. No, motivations are primal. They are related to the three biological imperatives that cannot be suppressed with impunity: to survive, to thrive and to reproduce. Any analysis of human motivation will ultimately reach this unyielding floor. This is a powerful tool because it permits you to predict human behavior (within limits obviously) and manipulate it. The more nimble you are in discerning bottom-line motives, the better you will skate around the pitfalls of societal living. You will quickly realize that what people say and what they do, are two entirely different things. What they say is meant to influence you or mislead you, and what they do is to satisfy their fundamental needs. This is why actions speak louder than words. You must become an expert in reading people between the lines and quickly uncover their deep motivations. This way you are better prepared to deal with them. The day you thoroughly understand that what motivates people is a net gain (unless they are psychotic!), the ingenious chess move is to find what that gain is. This whole discourse might sound a tad Machiavellian but it reflects simple reality.

- Your competitive position in society should be based on your capabilities. There is no point engaging the competitive minefield of society in a league where you can't possibly succeed or prosper. As already discussed in this book, there must be a proportionality between what you attempt and what is possible for you. The message, however, is not that you should be dissuaded from acceding to the highest peak, it is to be the best that you can be. Every part of you should be improved and thus heighten your competitive position. There is no substitute for excellence.

- Develop skills in conflict management. As soon as you approximate two or more individuals in the same environment, there is a potential for conflict. The root of this conundrum is when there are insufficient resources to satisfy the biological needs of everybody, be it food, shelter, love, money, etc., there will be a collision of wills and wants. This translates into a minefield of clashes. Quite apart from the theoretical basis of conflict, the simple observation of our world over the past few thousand years is enough to convince you that we live in a sea of conflict. Management of this everyday reality is crucial. Not only do you want to either win or resolve a conflict, you also want to know when a battle is not cost-effective. A chronic fatigue sufferer should not permit himself to be drawn into avoidable conflicts and to be unskilled in resolving them, when inevitable.

While clashes will involve, at one time or another, your parents, siblings, lovers, neighbors, workmates, competi tors, strangers, there is a common denominator. Most conflicts are utterly emotional in nature and have very little to do with logic. Even though we believe our respective positions to be logical, even though logic plays a paramount role in human communications, and even though logic is universally respected, it plays almost no role in generating or resolving human conflicts. Logic is, by and large, subjugated to a higher logic - that of emotions. This concept becomes clearer if one considers that emotions have evolved over billions of years to guide and safeguard the animal. Logic, a product of the incredible brain growth of the genus *Homo sapiens*, is a new kid on the block and not a primal determinant of human choices. When it comes to the fundamental biological imperatives of life (survival, thriving and reproduction), emotional dictates will override logic every time. Intellectual logic is foetal in its development; entirely understandable when one considers its recent arrival (~100,000 years) on the evolutionary timetable.

Since most conflicts arise because there is, in the final analysis, a threat to survival or reproductive opportunity, emotions will dominate the landscape. On that landscape, logic becomes hostage to personal interpretation. Personal interpretation will depend heavily on how the issue impacts on the person's life and it boils down to "judging" if the outcome is "good" or "bad" for the person in question.

If it was just a matter of judging good or bad, it would be a relatively simple matter to get at the core of the disputed matter. Not so. Our brain is metaphorically equipped with several layers of emotional lenses and filters that modify and diffract every bit of reality. External and internal information becomes colored, skewed, distorted and magnified with the net result that what is true and real for one individual may be quite the opposite for another. These emotional prisms grow with experience and are constantly reshaped. The reality of life as it is being progressively inscribed in your memory banks is assigned an emotional valuation.

Every experience in life reshapes our emotional valuation. When you attempt to penetrate your opponent's brain to accurately discern what makes him "tick," you will have to gain a glimpse of his experiential background:

past experience	ambitions
historical meaning	emotional sensitivity
cultural biases	judgement
religious meaning	race
vulnerabilities	prejudice
weaknesses	love
strengths	hate
knowledge	health status
education	sex
intelligence	age
philosophy	politics
financial status	social status

These serve to illustrate the many factors that impact on somebody's perception of what is "good" or "bad", beneficial or deleterious, and how one will judge the importance of an issue.

163

These add a fourth dimension to logic: an emotional one.

When one analyzes major social conflicts such as gun control, abortion and the death penalty, one can see how people, because of their different emotional valuation of the issue, can arrive at diametrically opposite views in spite of each displaying perfectly logical arguments.

It is crucial to understand these dynamics as they will permit you to accept differing opinions more readily and will give you ammunition to allay deep fears and anxieties that so often underlie the fierceness of a conflict.

There are different forms of conflict, each demanding a different technique to handle.

- Immutable options: when conflicting ambitions are chasing a single gainful conclusion. There are two wants and only one satisfactory result. If the options are intrinsically irreconcilable, they become immutable.

- Poor definition of the matter in dispute: overly sophisticated notions, unfamiliarity, ignorance, naivety and inexperience often lead to total confusion and cross-talk. People may be arguing about different things and not realize it.

- Imprecise language: it is so often the case that the whole raison d'etre of a conflict is a complete misunderstanding of what is meant or using imprecise language and misconstrued concepts.

- Divergent emotional valuations of the main elements of a conflict, as already discussed.

- Malevolence: I doubt that the conflict of World War II with Hitler was a case of imprecise definitions and blurry logic. There are conflicts whose internal dynamics are outright malevolence.

- Absence of logic: a conflict with an out-of-control psychotic individual will not yield to wise and logical deliberations.

Strategies of conflict management may then be constructed on the basis of the preceding discussion.

- Remove any ambiguity from the subject of conflict. Always question the original premise. Is everybody talking about the same thing? Be clear. Be focused. Don't wander. You can deal with tangential issues on another day.
- Elucidate the meaning of key words. Your meaning and someone else's might be two different things. A useful technique is to ask your dissenter to elaborate on what he or she means by certain key words. You may be surprised on how his or her perception is drastically different from yours. Avoid the Tower of Babel syndrome. Precise language and accurate thought delivery will go a long way towards solving irritating conflicts.
- The subjugation of logic to emotions: As discussed, the emotional valuation of an issue is complex, runs deep and will fuel hardening positions if not dealt with intelligently. Delve into your opponent's brain and sort out the dynamics of his personal valuation on the issue in question. Calm as many anxieties and satisfy as many needs as you can. With good insight and judicious adjustments in your battle position (so often at no cost), the gulf that initially separated your positions will narrow appreciably. Not infrequently, a conflict will spontaneously unravel once paralyzing fears, deep under the surface, are allayed.
- Immutable options, malevolence and aberrant logic: There are unfortunate circumstances where the conflict is so deeply-embedded in a concrete of irreconcilable positions that there is no hope of a satisfactory solution. The best-case scenario is a compromise, with a 50-50 movement on each side and let "bygones be bygones." In the absence of a civil compromise, the laws of the jungle take over. These laws still operate, like it or not. We are not that far removed from our vertebrate brethren. These natural laws are quite simple: if you are stronger than your opponent, advantaged strategically for one reason or another and

the putative clash offers a good cost-benefit ratio, you fight, destroy and win. If, on the other hand, you are weaker, disadvantaged and the struggle does not seem worth it, you abandon the fight and flee. There will be better days ahead.

A note of reassurance. A loss is not always what it seems to be. Life's fabric and human nature are so complex and riddled with twists and turns of fate that, not infrequently, a loss is a blessing in disguise. Conversely, a win may be tragic. At the very least, a loss is a powerful motivation to do better in the future, a valuable learning experience and another step towards the pinnacle of wisdom.

Skillful and efficient conflict resolution is an invaluable asset in the overall strategy to create social well-being.

- Avoid unproductive risk: There are risks that are perfectly legitimate. There is "le beau risque" in the French literature, and then there is stupid risk. High risk is an unnatural state. It implies a profound flaw in the process, an absence of subjugation to natural laws and the presence of smoke and mirrors camouflaging pure randomness. It is not acceptable to run one's life as a high-risk venture.

The individual suffering from chronic fatigue is very similar to the one whose financial capital is on the edge and who can be tipped into bankruptcy by the slightest change in wind direction. Can you conceive of this person betting his meager pennies at a Black Jack table, investing it in lottery tickets or trading futures options on the Chicago Exchange? Of course not. The person whose tolerance is diminished by fatigue should insulate himself from all high-risk schemes. He must avoid "stupid" risks. Examples:

- lack of car, home and disability insurance
- high-failure-rate business ventures
- short-term stock trading and most speculative derivatives of the stock market
- any gambling

166

- unsafe sex, substance abuse, reckless driving
- most contact sports and most sports disqualified for life insurance coverage (e.g. sky-diving)
- unhealthy diet, smoking, ignoring persistent physical symptoms or serious signs of illness (any blood loss, i.e. urine, stool, coughing)
- any crime

The list could go on but the above examples illustrate what foolhardy risks look like.

- Espouse a friendly attitude. We have all seen them. Tense, unsmiling, grumpy, discourteous boors who flail about with an attitude of uncaring arrogance and sow along their paths strife and hostility. These unfriendly characters are perceived as a threat and will never draw sympathy and true cooperation. They are doomed to be shunned and reviled. Not an ideal position in society.

The converse is a bonanza. Friendly people, at no cost to them, attract friendship, goodwill, cooperation and success. Yes, success, because at the end of the line a "friend" will get ahead of a "jerk." Always empathize, always smile and always display genuine respect for others.

MARRIAGE

A marital union is a microcosmic crucible of human relationships. How we handle this most fragile coupling and how we create a healthy family environment are decisive determinants of the fatigue sufferer's flourishment in home life. There is probably no more potent "devitalizer" and "enfeebler" than a toxic marriage. It alone can sap all your energy. Along with workplace conditions, the home environment will make or break you. The best investment a chronic fatigue sufferer can make is in his marriage or equivalent union.

When nature enjoins two distinct individuals for the purpose of fulfilling the imperatives of reproduction, it brings together partners with very different biological predispositions: different mating strategies, different nurturing intensities and styles, different personal needs, communication skills, emotional make-up, temperament, desires, agendas, likes and dislikes and so on, creating a fractious setting ripe for clashes. Some are inevitable but most are avoidable with proper forethought and circumspection.

STRATEGIES TO ENHANCE MARITAL WELL-BEING

Imagine a situation where you are forced to live with a stranger of the opposite sex on a permanent basis and it's your responsibility to make this relationship work. Leave romantic love out of the picture and devise a *modus operandi* that would give you the best possible chances of being happy in this constrained relationship.

You would probably dream up the following contrivance: the establishment of a warm companionship with all the advantages of friendship while permitting sufficient personal latitude to pursue individual, cherished ambitions.

The advantages of friendship are immense: security, personal validation, increased self-esteem, education, social support, healing, sounding board, confidence, love, loyalty, and recreation. Wouldn't it be a sorry loss to overlook a perfect opportunity to gain a close friend for life?

The respect for personal freedom is equally critical. We all have a unique chemistry, a unique spin on life. It is quite doubtful that significant happiness is achievable without this vital ingredient. Somehow there must be a compromise between the covenants of a relationship and person freedom. There lies the fulcrum where the marital equilibrium takes place.

(1) Children are the Exaltation of Marriage
Have many children! This is the raison d'etre of marriage. Children strengthen the marital bond, create a commonality of genetic interest and are a source of life-long happiness. Statistics support this contention : there is an inverse relationship between the num-

ber of children and the likelihood of divorce. With no children the divorce rate hovers around 40% and with one (25%), two (20%), and with three (3%), the rate diminishes dramatically. Other factors permitting, this would seem to be a productive approach.

(2) Cultivate the Qualities that Enhance Love

The qualities that were refined to attract your mate in the first instance should be bolstered and polished:

- physical attractiveness
- inner beauty
- genuine commitment
- dependability and security
- sincerity and kindness
- ambition and industriousness
- intelligence and knowledge
- mental and physical health
- generosity

(3) Weed Out Negative Behavior

Boorishness will most assuredly lead to the ruination of your marriage. Other effective destructive measures:

- excessive criticism
- defensiveness
- emotional withdrawal and retraction of love
- isolation and stone-walling
- abuse and violence
- deception and infidelity
- selfishness
- contempt and derogation

(4) Friendship Outlasts Passion

While we would all intuitively agree that friendship is a beneficial transformation within a marriage, in practice it is very problematic. The reasons for this are unclear. One could introduce a speculative notion. Friendship is a form of same-sex love that naturally bonds people who are similar biologically. Similarity of race, religion, education, culture, psychology, personality, temperament, ambitions, dreams and enjoyment of life creates an affinity. The broader the base of similarities, the stronger the relationship. Opposite sexes are not naturally attuned to an asexual friendship. Nature has programmed opposite sexes to be sexually attracted to each other, to reproduce and to nurture their offspring. This biological programming is quite different from the one for friendship. While friendship is based on similarity, romantic love is based on dissimilarity. The dissimilarity is an essential biological requisite for the genetic survival of the species.

The bottom line is that men and women are very different and therefore not well tuned to the casualness of friendship. This is a major stumbling block for a large number of marital unions.

How could one upgrade the state of friendship in a marriage? Emphasize the similarities between the partners and lessen the dissimilarities. One could draw up a list of all similarities and dissimilarities and devise practical means of activating the similarities while together and reserving any expression of dissimilarities when on personal freedom time. A simple example would be to enjoy what you both enjoy together, say watching movies or jogging, and when it's time to indulge in non-mutually satisfying activities, you do them separately, non-accusingly and on your own time. If you apply this philosophy to all segments of your life together, you will have made a giant step towards marital harmony.

(5) Respect Personal Freedom

Personal freedom within a romantic/sexual union is often misinterpreted. One suspects that the possessiveness and exclusivity of romantic love doesn't leave much room for wandering. And that's the problem. Personal freedom is interpreted as "wandering," diminished attraction or emotional withdrawal, or searching for someone "better." Personal freedom within a friendship is much easier to achieve, presumably because of the absence of romantic exclusivity.

To have personal freedom in a marriage, one must also allow his or her partner the same privilege. A one-way street will never work. Both partners must reach an understanding on personal freedom and build confidence through trust. When attained, the rest is "nuts and bolts." How much, when and where, is entirely discretionary and should only be worked out on an individual basis.

Regardless of the intricacies, the principle of granting each other personal freedom time is primordial. Spouses who cannot accept the legitimate pursuit of personal ambitions are courting potential disaster.

(6)   Eliminate the Irritants

We all harbor innumerable little habits which have no special meaning or purpose and are major irritants to our mates. They have no intrinsic value. Let's eliminate them.

Slurping, scratching, snorting, gurgling, burping, leaving the toilet seat up or down, not replacing the last leaf of the toilet paper roll, flicking channels when not alone, forgetting messages, talking on the phone too long, using certain expressions, not squeezing the toothpaste tube properly are but a few examples of petty misdeeds that drive spouses insane. Each partner should make a list of all the irritants, barter them in good faith and eradicate them! You will never miss them and you will both gain some measure of comfort.

(7)   Inject a Sense of Humor into Your Marriage

My wife tells me this is impossible. Her sense of humor is wonderful and mine is sick or aberrant (so true in marriages!). Ideally, we should be able to look at an event, size it up for what it is and emotionally deal with it in a favorable way. In other words, choose to interpret it in a humorous way. The value of humor is its capacity to reduce the emotional impact of an event by muting its physiological stress reaction.

How to develop a sense of humor and help your spouse do the same? Ameliorate your life as much as is humanly possible (it is difficult to have a sense of humor if you are starving or in jail) and train your mind to look at the humorous or bright side of life. Training means obstinate self-talk with the purpose of eventually developing psychological reflexes (new, improved neural circuits through plasticity) that slant your viewpoint towards humor.

Every day, pick an event of significance and reinterpret it in a light-hearted way. This daily training will gradually transform your perspective on life to a more lighthearted and up-beat one. So much of what transpires in life is out of our control. It might as well make us laugh rather than cry. External reality is not altered but your internal milieu is improved immeasurably.

If your partner or spouse joins you in this mind-set venture, the exercise doubly benefits the relationship.

(8) Share the "Scut" Work

If you can't afford to hire domestic help and disentangle your home life from "scut" work, then make sure it is shared fairly. There is nothing more demoralizing for a spouse than to feel exploited, abused and/or treated like a slave. It reflects a lack of respect and a lack of love. Nobody likes scut work and that is precisely why it should be shared fairly. Fairly, because equal is utopic. Depending on the weight of responsibilities on one spouse versus the other, scut work should be distributed in a mutually-agreeable fashion. Bite the bullet and stick to it. If you can't agree, flip a coin on a monthly basis.

(9) Manage Sex Common-Sensically

When the erotic phase of marriage wanes, the potential for misinterpreting this normal phenomenon rises dramatically. Sex is an integral part of a marital relationship and it is imbued with enormous symbolism. Very often, it is substituted as a barometer for love. As the sexual froth settles, a couple may feel their relationship is failing. Nothing could be further from the truth. It is exactly what it is: a normal phenomenon not to be misconstrued as a sign of deterioration.

The rules of the sexual game will vary enormously from one couple to the next. Hopefully, when the partner is selected at the outset, there isn't gross mismatching in this area. Part of the selection process should take into account the sexual landscape of your prospective mate. In any case, some form of accommodation should be reached to avoid two hovering rain clouds: making immoderate demands on the other in a covert fashion, converting an otherwise serene relationship into one stimulated by a constant irritating vigilance for "not again today." The other rain cloud is the miscalculation that less, or no sex, is equal to less, or no love.

The best approach is to put all the issues on the table, naked and raw. What you like or dislike, what you want and don't want and when and how often. Find a compromise and structure your sexual life accordingly. Forget spontaneity. Plan things consciously and eliminate the stress of uncertainty. It might seem to be a tad mechanical but it is a perfectly workable mode of operation. If you want an asexual marriage, have an asexual marriage if that is agreeable to both of you. If you want to swing from chandeliers every Saturday morning at 7:00 A.M., go for it!

The most difficult part is to expose your inner feelings. On this one, you have to bite the bullet, accept the risk and take a leap of faith. The ones who do will be immeasurably rewarded.

(10) Happiness is Contagious

If you concentrate on making yourself happy in the true biological sense, you will not only achieve personal well-being but your mate will be uplifted with you. If you are happy and fulfilled, you will be more beautiful, pleasant company, less conflicted, less prone to the degrading effects of stress, more generous, have a better sense of humor, and just simply be a more powerful human magnet. Your spouse will benefit from this and will likely emulate you. Happiness is contagious.

(11) Infidelity

Fidelity is largely a human idiosyncracy, although there are rare parallels in the animal world. Humanity has evolved a quasi-natural discriminatory possessiveness in the love arena. Marital unions, as currently practiced, cannot tolerate promiscuity. No matter how much you intellectualize this issue, emotionally, the absence of sexual exclusivity cannot be endured.

Every one of us has the capacity to fall in love with a variety of people and be sexually attracted to them. This is normal and it is the way biology is structured. This meets head-on with marital exclusivity. They cannot co-exist. A choice has to be made. The winner has to be marital exclusivity. How to cope? Sublimation! The energy accumulated by the preservation of marital exclusivity must be channeled into other compensatory endeavors. Only you can choose this endeavor. It could be anything from missionary work to climbing Mount Everest. The sky is the limit!

(12) Honour Human Values

Your spouse has an equal right to reach his/her full potential for happiness. He or she is a full-fledged member of the human race and deserves respect, a celebration of human dignity and all the benefits of honest communication to help resolve life's inevitable conflicts.

(13) Forgive and Forget

Forgiveness is a human quality that is the product of a deep visceral understanding of life's imperfections and frailties and the pure generosity of not exacting a price for an injurious affront. Why forgive? Because, on balance, there is more to gain than to lose. Life would be unbearable if we all kept a score card.

(14) Cut Loose

If your marriage is hell on earth no matter how hard you try, if the mismatch is irreconcilable, vent out the whole quandary in front of an impartial third party. If the ruination is confirmed by this third party, for example a marriage counselor, and the prognosis is dismal, cut loose and start all over again. Divorce might well be your last refuge for survival. A chronic fatigue sufferer will not likely survive a toxic marriage.

THE WORKPLACE

We spend one-quarter of our life in the workplace, a fiendish domain for the chronic fatigue sufferer. Work puts enormous demands on energy stores, emotional resilience and social subsistence. All three will have a tremendous impact on general health and the state of fatigue. As opposed to marriage, where the issue is primarily psychological well-being, here we are talking about naked survival. If you are too tired to work, if you are too physically impaired or psychologically drained to earn a living, you will perish (for all practical purposes). There is very little leeway for the chronically tired person. The right choices have to be made early and astutely.

(1) Right Choice of Career

The energy-impaired person obviously cannot even consider any work that entails intense physical labor or work which incorporates high mental stress levels. Forget construction work or traffic controlling, bypass the world of entertainment and ignore pressure-cooked adversarial professions (lawyer, politics, union leader, public relations etc). There are so many other more opportune careers that you will never miss the examples above. The exact choice is left to your personal discretion and visionary wisdom.

(2) Management of the Human Aspects of the Workplace

The work place presents rather singular problems. Not only does one have to cope with large numbers of individuals with differing personalities, temperaments and cultures, but one has to engineer a fine acrobatic balance between the need to cooperate and intrinsic competitiveness. Yes, you have to be a team player and at the same time, be highly competitive with your workmates.

Cooperation is the quintessential quality that is most cherished in the business world. It is the "make or break" issue that will, in large part, determine the comfort level of your position within an institution or a business. A team player is appreciated above all. A roguish, self-serving "in your face" type of style will quickly have you ostracized and this would only be the beginning of your misery.

Treat your co-workers as you would have them treat you. They are no better or worse than you and they have the same weaknesses, fears, vulnerabilities and their life struggle is just as intense. They also deserve to make a living. Respect for their human dignity will never lead you astray.

Always project an image of friendliness, always smile and be empathetic. It costs you absolutely nothing and you will be appreciated.

Competitiveness is the flip side of the coin but only superficially. One can be utterly friendly, respectful, cooperative and empathetic and be thoroughly competitive at the same time. Competition does not just mean that there is a winner and a loser as in a boxing match; it also means that you can be a better winner amongst many winners.

The two most important components of workplace competitive success is excellence and an entraining simultaneous net gain for the people connected to you. If you can master these two concepts, you will almost inevitably bubble up to the appropriate levels of the organization.

Excellence is a product of many factors. Knowledge is the key. Total knowledge. One should make a point of knowing everything there is to know about your trade and its related topics. Read everything you can in relevant areas and then read some more. Learn everything there is to know about your institution - its roots, its culture, its mission and, yes, its politics. The more you know, the better you will navigate the treacherous waters of the workplace. The importance of total knowledge cannot be over-emphasized. If you add to knowledge, hard work and passion, you will *de facto* be competitive.

While aggressiveness is seductive, totally American, and credited for the incredible wealth-producing feats of the business world, it is, in fact, an illusory approach. There is an important subtlety to grasp at this point. What has spurred success in business is not aggression where reaching the goal is achieved by crushing the enemy, breaking through walls of human resistance and climbing the ladder of success by using, as rungs, the heads of your competitors. No, the true secret of success is an incredible will to work hard, a concentrated effort to achieve, an understanding of the power of knowledge, the intelligence to find it and, finally and most pointedly, the insight to know that human values, human love, human cooperation and human generosity are pillars of the monument of success. In other words, competitiveness is not borne

176

out of crushing your enemies but, quite the contrary, by pulling them up with you to the heights of achievement. If you want to move up within an organization, you must not represent a threat but you must be perceived as a net gain for the individuals along the path and for the organization as a whole.

(3) Maximization of Income

It is as plain as the nose on one's face that maximal income is desirable. It is even more so in the handicapped individual who is prone to underperform or who may have to unexpectedly stop working because of illness or sheer exhaustion. The chronic fatigue sufferer should therefore orient himself towards the white-collar occupations and traditional professions in an attempt to carve out a more efficient income production. Average annual rates of income production is a good guide. Unfortunately, there is a *pari passu* greater competition for these prime jobs.

One approach to this conundrum is the exploitation of specialization. The more you know about a specific ultra-defined niche, the more valuable your service will be and, paradoxically, it will be faced with less competition. The same principle applies to a product. Another advantage of ultra-specialization is the greater flexibility of time management, which would allow you to introduce adequate periods of rest. A very important aspect of work selection.

(4) Adjust Your Work Output to Your Work Capacity: A Critical Balancing Act

Sometimes, less can mean more. There are some studies indicating that a professional may work fewer hours and still succeed. Sound like a pipe dream? It is perfectly doable. As an independent professional or businessman, there exists an inherent flexibility to downsize workload. Many large American corporations will allow customized work arrangements. A scaled-back work-week does slow an employee's career but it does not stop it. Better less and cope, than struggle and die. On some occasions, a reduced work schedule actually improves performance. If an employee is permitted to work at a comfortable pace, his long-term performance will be superior if only because of less breakdowns in productivity (sick leave etc).

Not all companies will sanction flexible or reduced work schedules and authorize rest periods but the climate is slowly changing. Alternative approaches could include working at home or settling for part-time employment.

(5) Build a Support Network

Fatigue is lessened and infinitely more supportable if there exists a rich social support network to buttress the unavoidable stumbles and tumbles. Friendship, amongst the others, is an invaluable asset. Family, spouse, friends, acquaintances, are all powerful pieces in the game of social chess. They should be cherished and the network should be developed to its maximum. Weigh the advantages of shared life experiences: sorrows are not as deep and prolonged, joys are magnified, boredom is mitigated, fatigue is tolerable, learning is amplified, errors are corrected, misperceptions are redirected, perspectives are put into focus, self-esteem is bolstered, opportunities for leisure are multiplied, and most pleasures in life are reinforced. Friendship is a treasure that must be earnestly nurtured.

In worst-case scenarios, where health or capacity to work falters, the support network provides a life-saving safety net.

CHAPTER 15
THERAPY OF CHRONIC FATIGUE IV:
STRIVE FOR MORAL EXCELLENCE

You may find it peculiar to include morality in a battle plan to combat fatigue. That might be because most people define morality in religious terms, which is a very narrow interpretation of what is a much deeper concept. Why should morality be restricted to the abeyance of religious laws? There are infinitely more imperatives in life than what this or that religion stipulates on. What was moral before mainstream religions were invented? What has guided humanity and its ancestors before religious inspiration exuded from an expanding brain mass and before religious thought could even be possible? One must dig much deeper to find true morality.

Morality is, indeed, a slippery concept. It is not an exclusively religious entity. Morality, in its broadest sense, assembles all the laws or regulations which must be embraced with compliant subjugation under the threat of some form of punishment. Table 15.1 summarizes the central features of morality and the main categories of laws which make it up.

Morality is activated by the deliberate choice of doing what is right or doing what is wrong. Right is what is "good" or beneficial to the person and wrong is what is "bad" or deleterious. In its most elemental state, morality is, in fact, a biological gate-keeper: natural laws have evolved over billions of years and our very existence is proof that they are effective. They are at the top of the totem pole and in any conflictual circumstance (where other sets of laws collide), they should dominate. Their track record is authenticated by our very existence.

Not as much can be said about political laws: these are man-made pieces of legislation that lamely attempt to manage society. If one looks back at the past few thousand years, with the enactment of millions of laws within dozens of different political systems, there is not much to cheer about. They are a testimony to the immaturity and flawed nature of the new kid on the block (in an evolutionary time frame). The enlarged brain of *Homo sapiens* is just beginning to flex its muscles.

Customs and mores are simply a cultural expression of natural laws and their mosaic reflect the diversity of our species.

Religious laws are difficult to fathom. The fundamental premise that a God exists, will liberate mankind from the clutches of evil and will transport us across the threshold of natural death into an eternal repository of unremitting peace and happiness is, to say the least, improbable if not downright ludicrous. In spite of this intellectual obstacle, humanity has spawned thousands of different religious systems, each with their own idiosyncratic laws. It is unclear which ones are genuine, significant, superior of simply capricious. Presumably the major religious structures have enough to offer their adherents to satisfy most human needs. The choice of religion becomes purely a matter of practicality or serendipity.

TABLE 15.1
MORALITY

LAWS	PURPOSE	YEARS OF EXISTENCE	PUNISHMENT
NATURAL LAWS	PROTECT THE BIOLOGICAL UNIT	BILLIONS	CELLULAR DISINTEGRATION ILLNESS, DEATH
CUSTOMS AND MORES	PROTECT THE SOCIAL UNIT	MILLIONS	DISCRIMINATION OSTRACIZATION
RELIGIOUS LAWS	SURVIVE DEATH	THOUSANDS	ETERNAL UN-HAPPINESS
POLITICAL LAWS	PROTECT SOCIETY	THOUSANDS	FINES IMPRISONMENT

Why ponder morality in the context of ameliorating chronic fatigue? Because its victim must observe a code of behavior which is pristine. To do this, he must fully grasp the breadth and consequences of the myriad of regulations that constrain his lifestyle. In this fashion, optimal choices can be made.

Moral laws should have weighting. They do not all have the same impact. One would not base health care on the Bible nor would one want to manage society with a textbook on thermodynamics. The different sets of rules in order of precedence for the fatigue sufferer are:

Natural laws > Customs and Mores > Political laws > Religious laws

Natural laws should dominate all decision-making. The bottom line should always be what is biologically beneficial. Natural laws are based on our biological nature and are the consequences of a long evolutionary process that has implacably rejected the

181

unworkable, the weak and the incompetent. This is not a system of laws that is created by, and imposed by an outside agent. They are inherent, intrinsic and *de facto* "moral." After four billion years of weeding out unsuccessful ventures, the system of natural laws is as good as it gets. To change the rules now would be sheer folly.

The fundamental thrust of natural laws is the multitude of processes that regulate the function of our basic unit of life, the cell, and the biological imperatives of survival, thriving and reproduction. The adverse consequences of non-observance of these intrinsic rules are cellular or organ dysfunction with the attendant pain, illness and exacerbation of a state of fatigue. Remember that fatigue is a biological pacesetter for cellular function and will play a large role in expressing the downside of unnatural or immoral behavior. The chronic fatigue sufferer must follow natural laws to the letter or face the consequences: greater fatigue. The ultimate repercussion of neglecting natural imperatives is death itself. No other system of laws can supplant this one.

HOW TO COMPLY WITH NATURAL LAWS

Natural laws are difficult to decipher and interpret. Mother nature does not reveal her secrets very easily. The main obstacle to fully abiding by nature's rules is our own ignorance of biology and other life sciences. Slowly, over centuries, this mass of unenlightenment is eroding and mankind proportionately benefits.

The observance of natural laws depends on knowledge and skills in monitoring the feedback information that guides it. Knowledge is a pre-requisite. One must learn as much as is humanly possible about biology, the human body in particular, anthropology, psychology, sociology, philosophy and the physical sciences. You can never learn too much. Every increment in knowledge nourishes the wisdom of decision-making and approximates one's total health to an optimal state.

The second aspect of complying with natural laws, is the ability to read feedback information from the choices made. How does nature tell us if what we are doing is right or wrong, good or bad? It tells us by altering our state of happiness. Happiness is not an emotion. It is a fundamental biological state of contentment that reacts to the health or wholesomeness of very single part of the body and "soul." Whatever detracts from health or a biologically wholesome state will degrade happiness or cause unhappiness; what enhances it will promote happiness. This state of happiness becomes an extremely useful barometer of success in observing natural laws. If whatever you are doing enhances your state of genuine happiness, you are on the right track.

BE A LAW-ABIDING CITIZEN

Once you have acquired the wisdom of rigorous compliance with natural laws, do you ignore or neglect the others? Not at all. The last thing a chronic fatigue sufferer should do is side-step them. There is way too much stress, grief and risk in breaking the rules of society. In any case, they are, by and large, beneficial as they protect the public and oil this huge apparatus of communal living. If you don't respect customs and mores, there will be inevitable discrimination and ostracization. If you break political laws (laws passed by legislators), you will be either financially penalized or imprisoned. This certainly does not improve fatigue.

Religious laws are a different kettle of fish. They do not apply to nature or society. How could they possibly apply to society when there are literally hundreds of religious systems with conflicting and idiosyncratic rules? The history of religious governance (theocracy) is a blood-stained attestation to its total unsuitability as a social manager. Religious adherence and devotion is an utterly personal endeavor. It should be kept strictly private. If you have faith, regardless of your specific religious affiliation, follow your leader's teachings, moral tenets and imbue yourself with the messages of hope and love that are fundamental to most mainstream religions.

A strong religious conviction may well be a highly advantageous attribute to the chronic fatigue sufferer. Religious faith yields remarkable psychological benefits. In fact, for the downtrodden or victims of life's harshness, it can literally be life-saving. One should not belittle the potential gain of full spiritual exaltation. The person, in exile from a full energetic life, will find refuge in God, the ultimate source of strength and vitality. If one truly believes, it will happen.

CHAPTER 16
THERAPY OF CHRONIC FATIGUE V:
THE MANAGEMENT OF ENERGY

The state of fatigue, the consequence of a dysequilibrium between energy supply and demand, is best managed by a meticulous accounting of the organisms's disbursements. A serious challenge against this enemy cannot be mounted without a full exploitation of efficiency measures, the elimination of energy wasters, the adoption of natural energy boosters and setting the most appropriate pace for one's comings and goings.

ERADICATE ENERGY WASTERS

There should be a constant review of one's daily stirrings to pinpoint the countless acts typifying energy wasters, either because they are unproductive or associated with emotional distress. Emotional distress is a supreme energy waster and deserves particular attention.

Common Energy Wasters:

- artificial time limits
- time pressure
- hurrying
- lack of organization
- talking instead of listening
- messiness
- uncomfortable posture
- fidgeting
- overeating (the energy consumed by digesting is considerable)
- heavy clothing
- heavy briefcase
- perfectionism and obsessive compulsive behaviour
- stress
- revenge or vengefulness
- sleeping pills
- tranquilizers
- cigarette smoking, alcoholism
- too hot or cold environment
- absence of a warm-up for demanding tasks
- remote location of everyday-use appliances
- scouring around for a location instead of asking for directions
- comparison shopping by foot instead of by phone
- argumentative attitude
- incessantly re-phoning instead of leaving a message to call back

Systematically weed out these and any other energy waster. You will be stockpiling vital energy stores for what you really want to accomplish.

EMBRACE ENERGY BOOSTERS

Let's make it very clear at the outset that there is no pure play in this realm of fatigue. There is no safe, useful or effective booster of "physical" energy. Forget about the magic elixirs, the wonder herb and the assorted power drinks. They are not effective. Don't even consider the use of potent pharmacologic agents such as amphetamines. They are counter-productive and potentially dangerous. The healthy well-maintained human body cannot be supercharged to increase energy production beyond its specifications. You cannot perpetually overdrive biochemical reactions or metabolic processes. It is true that an inadequate nutrition will starve the machinery and lead to fatigue, but the converse does not apply. No amount of "super-feeding" with any nutritional ingredient will boost the chronic fatigue sufferer. No iron, no vitamins, no electrolyte, no carbohydrate "bomb," no "natural" product will help. When it seems to, you are probably witnessing a placebo reaction.

The only known natural energy boosters are psychological. You will readily recognize them because at one time or another you have experienced their uplifting effect.

- fulfilling work
- success
- enhanced self-esteem
- positive attitude
- optimism
- happiness
- love
- religious exaltation
- motivation

A word of caution. The above are doubled-edged. Indulge excessively and they turn on you and aggravate fatigue. There must exist a tempered indulgence sprinkled with aggressive self-restraint. Just like spices, to complete a culinary masterpiece.

BE EFFICIENT

The proposition is straightforward. Get from point A to point B while consuming less energy. Same result, less fatigue. Efficiency measures are a boon for fatigue sufferers.

Faster should not be confused with more efficient. Quite the opposite.Speed exacts a premium. Not unlike a car engine that guzzles disproportionate amounts of gasoline at high speeds, the human body imposes a heavy tax for celerity.

Most efficiency measures cost money. This highlights another aspect of the life of the fatigue sufferer: money is crucial, much more than for a healthy person.

Examples of efficiency measures follow:

- pay for services that you do not wish to do yourself or that simply cannot be tolerated energetically: house cleaning, house repairs, grass mowing, landscaping, gardening, snow removal
- dry-cleaning clothes instead of washing, drying and ironing
- ready-made meals instead of cooking, cleaning and dishwashing
- critical positioning of everyday-use appliances to reduce walking distances
- milking the efficiency gains created by modern technology: washer and dryers, dishwashers, mixers, food processors, microwave ovens, computers, computerized time management, electric garage door openers, self-propelled grass mowers, etc.
- let your fingers do the walking: do your comparison shopping by phone or on-line (internet), not by foot
- do on-line shopping and have it delivered to your door
- avoid traffic hours
- if you have two homes, double-up on sundries to avoid packing and unpacking
- ask for directions instead of scurrying around
- learn from a pro instead of fumbling around with self-teaching
- double-tasking - a classic: open your mail on the John
- cluster errands: accumulate your chores and do them all in one sitting with an efficient sequence (shopping, bank-

ing, appointments etc)
- when shopping for food, buy in large quantities with home delivery; this way you reduce the number of shopping sprees
- when cooking a meal, make extra for tomorrow's lunch
- when cooking certain foods, make large quantities for several meals (soups, sauces etc)
- be super-organized and plan ahead; make lists
- be neat
- delegate as much as possible
- when attempting to reach someone by phone, leave a message instead of incessantly re-phoning: let them find you. Leave an intriguing message. That should accelerate the return call.
- discover short-cuts: re-examine your routines and assess them for maximum efficiency
- self-help devices: tools with enlarged handles, jar openers, reachers
- wear light clothing, carry a light purse or briefcase
- unpleasant tasks should be "routinized" and done "automatically" to remove the emotional content
- do everything "well" the very first time around; you don't want to constantly correct yourself
- buy the very best you can afford at the outset; it turns out to be less trouble in the long run and, in fact, cheaper
- always "warm-up" before attempting a difficult task: the body is more efficient when "warm"

PACING AND MATCHING

The person who is prone to fatigue is responsible for finding the perfect equilibrium between energy supply and demand and the appropriate amount of rest for full recuperation. Nobody else can prescribe it. By a process of trial and error, one usually discovers this critical balance. Pacing is the crucial tactic. Finding the right rhythm that best fulfils the demands of your personal universe without imposing punishing fatigue is an art that only you can master.

Pacing implies the absence of expensive peaks of activity. One must avoid the push-crash sequence as it is very damaging from a fatigue point-of-view. This would be the equivalent of fartlek training where an athlete regularly inserts segments of very high intensity sprinting within his running routine. Sudden explosions of energy consumption are prohibitively expensive for the fatigue sufferer and should be eliminated altogether.

Matching refers to doing difficult or unpleasant tasks at a time of day when one is generally the strongest or most energetic. You reserve these chores for when you are feeling your best.

Practice relaxation techniques and time critical napping sessions when you feel they are the most productive. For example, the post-lunch period is often a time we naturally slump and is generally a good time to nap. Relaxation techniques are a boon particularly when one is facing stressful duties. A useful technique entails finding a perfectly comfortable body position to then sequentially relax each muscle of the body and maintain this state of total body looseness for 10 to 15 minutes. Along with the physical unwinding, one adds a complete blanking of the mind. If not possible, then blank out, at the very least, the thoughts specifically related to the stressful event being experienced. When available, a body massage is heavenly.

Rest does not only mean "doing nothing". Leisure activities play a very important role in the lives of chronic fatigue sufferers. Join a swim club, take up bowling, curling, billiards, watch movies or simply go for long walks and admire nature or the snow crackling under your feet. Read romance novels, listen to music, vegetate, indulge in a hobby, sew, watch TV etc. The possibilities are endless. Stick to what you enjoy and stay away from competitive activities or overly-demanding ones, physically or intellectually (e.g. chess).

With knowledge and wisdom, anybody can effectively manage their energy stores no matter how meager they are.

Dr. Claude R. Maranda

CHAPTER 17
THERAPY OF CHRONIC FATIGUE VI: MEDICAL THERAPY

Any person afflicted with an unnatural burden of fatigue should develop a strong relationship with a physician, a most invaluable resource in the battle against incapacitating tiredness. He has the expertise to rule out significant medical problems, to refer you to the appropriate specialist for specific problems, to give you valuable advice and to treat you either psychotherapeutically or pharmacologically when indicated.

PSYCHOTHERAPY

Psychotherapy is not especially useful for pure cases of low energy or easy fatiguability. It is not a psychiatric illness or a neurosis as such. However, to the extent that psychological dysfunction may be contributing to the condition, psychotherapy may be helpful. Most physicians will stick to elementary support therapy, primarily reassurance

191

and encouragement. Group therapy may be very helpful, if available in your area. It is very reassuring to commiserate with similarly-afflicted fellow human beings and is highly consoling when the condition exacerbates. Wonderful insights may be shared and the whole process can be singularly educational.

PHARMACOTHERAPY

Drug therapy plays a minor role in the management of idiopathic fatigue. Certainly, specific medical conditions can be treated effectively. In some cases, cured; in others, palliated.

Examples:
- hyperthyroidism can be cured by anti-thyroid medications, radiotherapy or surgery
- chronic inflammatory disorders can be improved with corticosteroids and/or immuno-suppressive therapy
- chronic viral illnesses such as AIDS can be palliated with anti-viral medications
- allergies can be greatly improved by antihistamines and desensitization therapy

When a depressive illness seems to be at the root of the problem, or secondary, as the consequence of incessant fatigue, therapy with anti-depressants is indicated. The most effective and well-tolerated, are the ones classified as serotonin-re-uptake inhibitors. These have been discussed in the section on depression.

In circumstances where anxiety is a significant aggravator of fatigue, the judicious use of anxiolytics may be very helpful. Frequently used drugs are the benzodiazepines such as alprozolam, clonazepam and lorazepam. This form of therapy should be closely supervised by your physician, not because it is risky (it is quite safe medically), but because there is a high risk of dependency. These drugs are very addictive psychologically. Once addicted, the process is difficult to reverse.

Insomnia is such a potent progenitor of fatigue that it requires special mention. When natural means of therapy are ineffective, there is a place for sleeping pills. They are strictly for the short-term alleviation of an exceptional stress or ailment. They too, are very addictive and will readily install themselves as unyielding dictators. Sleeping pills may well be the most abused medication in America. The medical profession has not been particularly effective in stemming this abuse. In the long run, meticulous sleep hygiene is more effective than sleeping pills.

Another problem with sleeping pills is their negative impact on the quality of sleep. Certain stages of sleep are adversely affected. The result is incomplete restoration and a paradoxical worsening of chronic fatigue. Sleeping pills are definitely not a long-term solution for anything in general and for fatigue in particular.

The pharmacotherapy of illnesses, not directly causative of severe dominant fatigue, is still somewhat useful when a debilitating symptom secondarily aggravates or initiates a fatigue state. For example, chronic pain for any reason will frequently devitalize the patient just on the basis of protracted physical stress. I have seen cases of Herpes Zoster, commonly known as shingles, where the constant severe pain will literally 'waste" away the victim.. Some individuals lose up to forty pounds in weight and are basically bed-ridden from loss of energy. Pain control by pharmacological means would obviously be helpful in such cases.

Analgesic drugs run the gamut from a simple non-anti-inflammatory analgesic such as acetaminophen to innumerable non-steroidal anti-inflammatory drugs such as aspirin, ibuprofen, naproxen and steroidal anti-inflammatory drugs such as cortisone. The latter are strictly prescription drugs because of the serious side-effects with long-term use. Finally, for extreme pain, morphine and its many derivatives (codeine, oxycodone, hydromorphine) are indicated but only as a last resort. They are highly addictive.

Occasionally, anti-depressant and anti-convulsant drugs are helpful in special types of pains such as lancinating neuritic pains. Neuritic pains are notorious for provoking a state of chronic fatigue because they interfere so much with proper sleep.

Migraine sufferers are occasionally reduced to a state of exhaustion. Beta-blockers, most often used for hypertension and angina pectoris will often be quite effective in this condition. Others may respond extremely well to a new medicine called Imitrex.

There is a group of men and women, more frequently women, who suffer from incessant tiredness and have a low blood pressure. It is not clear if there is a cause and effect relationship or if they are simply associated. This association is surprisingly common. It may be worthwhile, in selected cases, to attempt to raise the blood volume so as to raise the blood pressure. High salt and high water intake might help or, in exceptional cases, where the low blood pressure is overtly symptomatic (i.e. fainting spells) the addition of a mineralocorticoid drug (Florinef) should be effective. This drug induces salt and water retention from the kidneys, increases blood volume and in this fashion raises blood pressure. This therapy is only indicated when the blood pressure is seriously low. A theoretical alternative therapy would be the usage of vasoconstrictive drugs. By increasing peripheral vascular resistance they raise the blood pressure. For a host of medical reasons, these drugs are hopelessly ineffective and impractical. Support hose might be helpful in reducing venous pooling in the upright position and help maintain an adequate blood pressure.

Experimental drug therapies are far in between and few in numbers.
- there is Ampligen, a nucleic acid product, which stimulates interferons (a family of immune response modifiers) that has some anti-viral activity and may be helpful for a subset of victims of the Chronic Fatigue syndrome
- testosterone derivatives such as dehydroepiandrosterone may be helpful in relieving the asthenia of waning testosterone levels in ageing males. They could soften the impact of the so-called male menopause (very controversial)
- other anabolic steroids (as the ones illegally used by certain athletes) may play a role in cases of illnesses associ-

ated with wasting and cachexia
- human growth hormone could possibly play a minor role in revitalizing the elderly who are the single largest group of chronic fatigue sufferers

Amphetamines are potent stimulants which, on a short-term basis, will explosively increase energy levels. Cerebral stimulants such as Ritalin and Cyclert could theoretically improve a state of fatigue transiently. Because of their ineffectiveness in the long-term, their toxicity and addictive potential, they are not indicated in any shape or form for the treatment of chronic fatigue. In any case, because of their illicit use for chemical "highs", they are a highly restricted class of drugs.

CHAPTER 18
ALTERNATIVE THERAPIES:
FACT OR FICTION?

Sufferers of chronic fatigue are particularly vulnerable to the exaggerated claims of untested and unproven forms of "alternative" treatments. They are desperate because, for them, life is a painful torment. Constant fatigue is frankly discouraging and will often lead to an imprudent embrace of any false prophet or any false cure. This is perfectly understandable. Any illness which cannot be handled effectively by the medical profession is fodder for marginal and sham therapies.

Whole industries have been erected to meet the needs of these people. Everything under the sun has, at one time or another, been promoted as a magical cure for whatever ails you. Unfortunately, the track record of these alternative and "fringy" types of therapies is not good. The facts resonate like a broken record: every single time one or the other of these magical remedies is scientifically tested with well-designed double- blind studies, they flounder under the weight of scientific rigor. It is indeed an extremely rare "alternative" treatment claim that will withstand the enlightenment of rigorous scientific scrutiny.

No amount of reality testing discourages the promoters. As soon as you discredit one, five more appear on the landscape. It is absolutely not cost-effective or even possible to properly study all these claims. They are simply too numerous.

A survey of what is "pushed" on the marketplace will be very helpful to the chronic fatigue sufferer so that he may be forewarned.

ALTERNATIVE THERAPIES OF A PHYSICAL NATURE

They include:
- Acupuncture: an ancient Chinese method of healing by inserting fine needles into specific points on the body.
- Chiropractic: manipulation of the spine to correct a misalignment for ailments that range from back pain to indigestion to insomnia.
- Polarity Therapy: balancing energy to restore the natural healing flow. Done by manipulations of specific points on the body leading to a more vital body and clearer mind.
- Hypnotherapy: the induction of a trance where the hynotized may have enhanced memory, greater suggestibility and transference from the therapist.
- Neurotherapy: biofeedback therapy which provides information to a person regarding one or more physiological process in an effort to enable functions that normally operate outside consciousness
- Touch Therapy: a variety of bodily strokings putatively therapeutic
- Aromatherapy: the use of fragrant oils to improve general health and relieve miscellaneous conditions
- High colonic enemas: presumably to cleanse the body of noxious substances originating from the colon.
- Yoga: exalted meditation in specific body positions
- Tai'Chi: a gentle form of muscular conditioning originating from China

- Music Therapy: the use of music to induce a therapeutic state.

The common denominator of all the physical manipulations is the "jogging" of one sensory organ or the other to heal whatever they are purported to heal. The following list catalogues the different sensory organs involved:

- deep touch: polarity therapy, chiropractic, colonic enemas
- superficial touch: acupuncture and touch therapy
- positional sense: yoga
- sense of smell: aromatherapy
- sense of hearing: music therapy, hypnotherapy
- sense of vision: hypnotherapy
- inner sense: neurotherapy

These sensory manipulations, with atypical stimuli, are, evidently, purported to induce a beneficial physiological state.

The range of physiological effects is rather limited: there is some psychological soothing which is primarily a placebo reaction, some relaxation of muscle and some element of pain control possibly through the release of endorphins in the brain. This just about sums it up. There is no plausible reason for sensory stimulation of any kind to have significant therapeutic effect in the setting of true pathology.

What the practitioners of these various therapeutic modalities fail to realize is the highly specialized mission of sensory organs. They are not "healing" switches to be turned on or off by a magician. They are organs that tranduce stimuli from the external world (light, sound waves, chemicals, physical deformaties) into an electrochemical signal transported by peripheral nerves into the central nervous system for perception and learning. What in the world this physiological function could possibly have to do with healing anything is below the credibility bar of anybody with minimal scientific knowledge or common sense.

The bottom line is that none of these treatment modalities have ever been proven effective for the relief of chronic fatigue.

ALTERNATIVE THERAPIES OF A CHEMICAL NATURE

Here, there is a mixed bag of substances, both natural and un-natural, that have been touted as panaceas for all that ails human-ity, including fatigue. You have all witnessed the marketing frenzy feverishly pushing the latest energizer. These are:
- dietary supplements
- multi-vitamin preparations
- minerals
- adenosine monophosphate
- coenzyme Q-10
- germanium
- glutathione
- iron
- magnesium sulfate
- melatonin
- NADH
- selenium
- L-tryptophan
- vitamins B_{12}, C and A
- zinc
- herbal preparations: astralogens, forage, seed oil, fromelain, comfrey, echinacea, garlic, gingko biloba, gin-seng, primrose oil, guercetin, St. John's Wort, Shiitake mushroom extract, and more.

The problem with all these substances is that:
1. Their effects are not biologically plausible.
2. In some preparations, one does not know what is actually being ingested.
3. Some of these substances are harmful in large dosages
4. The long term safety of large doses of even natural sub-stances cannot be guaranteed.
5. Most are largely untested.
6. Almost none have scientifically proven efficacy
7. Serious physicians are highly skeptical of their benefits

8. Professional medical associations do not officially endorse them.
9. The motive is economic

These "chemical" ingestants fall into two categories. One is the group of substances that are found naturally in the body and play an essential metabolic role such as minerals, vitamins and certain enzymes. Why should it be in any way therapeutic to ingest large "pharmacologic" doses of any of these natural substances? Once you have crossed the threshold of having a sufficient supply for the body's needs, there is no biological bonus to take more. If one examines carefully the dynamics of a biochemical reaction, one would easily understand how substrate overabundance does not accelerate the reaction or lead to more product. What actually happens biologically is this: when there is an oversupply of substrate, it is either stored, excreted by the kidneys or (gastrointestinal tract) or accumulates in the tissues where it could be harmful. For example, an excess of carbohydrates will be stored in glycogen, an excess of fat in adipose tissue, an excess of vitamins is excreted externally by the kidneys or stored in organs such as the liver and skin, and an excess of minerals is generally excreted by the kidneys. An oversupply of any natural substance simply does not beget "more product" or "more effect." It is very much like a car engine. The body will consume exactly what it needs to perform its task. Adding more gasoline in the fuel tank of a car will not increase the work of the engine. It will only accumulate in the tank in reserve. Overfilling the tank will only lead to overflow and spillage. In an oversimplified fashion, the body's biochemical engines work very much the same way.

As far as the unnatural substances go and here we refer to all the exotic herbal preparations and assorted substances that are not normally found in the body, the matter in question is even more serious. Here we are asked to believe that this totally foreign molecule floating around in our body will magically couple itself to our cellular receptors, invade our most intimate biochemical processes and alter our neuro-transmitter substances to improve or cure the ailing system!

This scenario is about as probable as creating gold by mixing sand and asphalt. If you believe that a random non-specific "chemical" effect (and that is assuming that the effect is not noxious) will make you more energetic, stronger and more intelligent, then you believe in Santa Claus.

Beyond the biological implausibility of these magic potions, one has to be very concerned about their potential harmful effects on the unsuspecting consumer. If you have any doubts about this, simply consider the fact that even perfectly natural and wholesome chemicals such as vitamins can be very toxic in large doses. The following selected list will give you an eye-opening glimpse as to what can result if you "take too much of a good thing." Now, imagine what could happen with totally foreign chemicals.

Vitamin and Mineral Excess	Illness
vitamin D	hypercalcemia
vitamin A	cerebral edema
vitamin E	headaches
vitamin K	coagulopathy
vitamin B6	neuropathy
vitamin C	renal stones
nicotinic acid	flushes
iron	diabetes
zinc	gastric ulcer
copper	cirrhosis
manganese	psychosis
cobalt	cardiomyopathy
chromium	renal failure
selenium	hair loss
fluoride	pneumonitis
calcium	renal stones
magnesium	neuropathy
sodium	hypertension
potassium	paralysis
iodine	hyperthyroidis

Let's face it. Most of these so-called "natural" products are untested, unproven, not certified as safe and they are as likely to be truly efficacious as holding a winning lottery ticket. Don't even bother! Divert the money to your favorite research fund.

You might ask, what about drugs that physicians prescribe every day? Aren't they foreign chemicals, unnatural substances? Don't they improve the health status of a sick person? Yes, but there is a fundamental difference. Drugs do not improve or increase the performance of a cell or an organ. Absolutely not. They cause a physiological abnormality, a diminishment of function, a stimulation of unnatural biochemical reactions and they interfere with normal biological processes. Yes, they absolutely do. They are poisons, but benign poisons that have a specific purpose. They neutralize another abnormality. In this way, they benefit the sick. An example will clarify this pivotal point.

Congestive heart failure is an increasingly prevalent condition. It is due to the diminished strength of contraction of the heart muscle. The most common cause is coronary atherosclerosis, which, by occluding coronary arteries, interrupts blood flow. The portions of the heart muscle that are thus deprived of oxygen and nutrients, die, and are replaced by scar tissue. A weakened heart cannot sustain the circulation adequately and this inadequacy triggers numerous physiological compensatory mechanisms. Clinically, we see accumulation of fluid causing congestion of the lungs and extremities, a rapid heart beat stimulated by the sympathetic nervous system and a decreased blood pressure.

Drugs are very useful in this condition, but not because they benefit normal physiological function. No, because they induce cellular aberrations which, fortuitously, benefit the organism. We use water pills, diuretics, to eliminate the fluid that congest the patient. This drug diffuses to the kidney, attaches itself to cells of the renal tubule, and interferes with its normal ability to absorb sodium and water. This drug-induced paralysis of normal tubular function leads to excretion of sodium and water and, in this fashion, counteracts the body's compensatory salt and water-retaining efforts.

202

We also use Digoxin, a heart muscle stimulant, that increases the force of contraction. Well, it doesn't do this by improving cellular physiology; it does it by poisoning the cell. It inhibits enzymes ($Na^+ K^+$ pump ATPase) which alters the electrochemical gradient of the muscle cell and permits entry of abnormally large quantities of calcium. This is highly unnatural, but the large quantities of calcium increase the power of muscle contraction. Another poison that has a beneficial overall effect.

Other drugs that are useful in this context are what are commonly called ACE inhibitors. They suppress certain enzymes which alter the levels and activity of several hormones, the net effect of which lead to an unnatural relaxation of the vasculature. This effect counter-balances the vasoconstrictive hormones that the heart failure stimulates. Again, an abnormal, un-physiologic state to neutralize another one.

Finally, beta-blockers are occasionally used in congestive heart failure. They block receptors on the heart muscle cell to diminish the constant bombardment of the heart by stress hormones, catecholamines. These latter hormones are toxic when their levels are too high. Thus, an induced anomaly to counteract a pathological state.

The point of this discussion is to highlight an elemental fact: foreign chemicals that are introduced into the body do not benefit normal physiology. In the instance of standard pharmacotherapy, drugs induce precise cellular functional aberrations with a mission of counteracting another aberration. In a healthy individual, there is no role for such chemical ruses. It simply does not work. The upshot is that the whole array of herbal, "natural", exotic and mega-vitamin concoctions is simply irrelevant on two counts: if you are truly sick, you need standard medical therapy and, if you are not, you don't need anything.

The conclusion to this long-winded dissertation is that your state of disabling fatigue will not be improved one iota with any of the physical or chemical "alternative" forms of pseudo-medical therapy that are aggressively marketed in our society.

ALTERNATIVE THERAPIES OF A PSYCHOLOGICAL NATURE

What about quick-fix psychotherapy? Some claim their particular "technique" or "psycho-intervention" will cure your phobias, your addictions and your fatigue. From "thought field therapy" to browsing through your childhood experiences for abuse, to a medley of "mood therapies", the fatigue sufferer will be bombarded with spectacularly unproven forms of quick-fix psychotherapies. How to protect yourself? Only accept the opinion of a certified psychiatrist with a pristine reputation and therapies that are officially sanctioned by either the American Medical Association or the American Psychiatric Association. When faced with exotic virtual-reality forms of voodoo therapy, and they have the feel of garbage, then you are probably dealing with garbage. Avoid these like the plague. Your medical care is much too important to leave in the hands of dream-merchants and snake-oil peddlers.

EPILOGUE

Fatigue is the universally-experienced inner sense of an ill-feeling signaling the presence of an imbalance between energy demand and energy supply. This imbalance in a healthy state is the result of excessive work and in an unhealthy state, dysfunction of the machinery supporting energy metabolism. In either instance, fatigue is a biological pace-setter whose mission is the protection of physiological systems against the damaging effects of chronic overwork. It should be regarded as an important control mechanism to be respected religiously.

The sense of frustration which regularly attends incapacitating fatigue should be tempered by the knowledge that it is, in a certain way, your friend, a most opportune friend. The problem is not fatigue itself; it is only a sign of a problem. Excessive fatigue gives you two critical pieces of information: either you are working too hard or there is something wrong with you, both in a very broad sense. It is then your responsibility to react appropriately.

This biological alarm signal provides you with an incredible opportunity, an opportunity to turn your life around and improve it beyond your most optimistic expectations. Let fatigue guide you to a more effective and happy life. You can modify your lifestyle by introducing a delicate equilibrium between its crucial components, you can improve your general health immmeasurably and you can wisely and astutely navigate the treacherous waters of society. All in all, you can optimize every single aspect of your life.

The individual who captures the message emanating from the pages of this book will not only make peace with fatigue, but will have conquered it by turning it on its head: a provident incitement to be the best you possibly can.

The crucial steps have been clearly delineated in this book:

- weed out pathological factors, be they physical, psychological or environmental
- upgrade your physical health to its utmost
- enhance psychological well-being to its maximum
- discover moderation and the magical equilibrium of life
- know yourself and adjust your goals accordingly
- be street-smart
- be realistic
- love yourself

If you follow this humble advice, fatiguability will be transformed into a blessing in disguise.

Dr. Claude R. Maranda

Dr. Claude R. Maranda

Coping With Fatigue

Dr. Claude R. Maranda

Coping With Fatigue